Diversity in Urology

Editor

TRACY M. DOWNS

UROLOGIC CLINICS
OF NORTH AMERICA

www.urologic.theclinics.com

Editor-in-Chief
KEVIN R. LOUGHLIN

November 2023 • Volume 50 • Number 4

ELSEVIER

1600 John F. Kennedy Boulevard • Suite 1800 • Philadelphia, Pennsylvania, 19103-2899

http://www.theclinics.com

UROLOGIC CLINICS OF NORTH AMERICA Volume 50, Number 4
November 2023 ISSN 0094-0143, ISBN-13: 978-0-443-13037-3

Editor: Kerry Holland
Developmental Editor: Nitesh Barthwal

Urologic Clinics of North America (ISSN 0094-0143) is published quarterly by Elsevier Inc., 360 Park Avenue South, New York, NY 10010-1710. Months of issue are February, May, August, and November. Business and Editorial Offices: 1600 John F. Kennedy Blvd., Suite 1800, Philadelphia, PA 19103-2899. Periodicals postage paid at New York, NY and additional mailing offices. Subscription prices are $415.00 per year (US individuals), $832.00 per year (US institutions), $100.00 per year (US students and residents), $473.00 per year (Canadian individuals), $1040.00 per year (Canadian institutions), $100.00 per year (Canadian students/residents), $546.00 per year (foreign individuals), $1040.00 per year (foreign institutions), and $240.00 per year (foreign students/residents). Foreign air speed delivery is included in all *Clinics* subscription prices. All prices are subject to change without notice. **POSTMASTER:** Send address changes to *Urologic Clinics of North America*, Elsevier Health Sciences Division, Subscription Customer Service, 3251 Riverport Lane, Maryland Heights, MO 63043. **Customer Service: 1-800-654-2452 (US). From outside the United States, call 1-314-447-8871. Fax: 1-314-447-8029. E-mail: JournalsCustomerServiceusa@elsevier.com (for print support)** and **JournalsOnlineSupport-usa@elsevier.com (for online support).**

Reprints. For copies of 100 or more, of articles in this publication, please contact the Commercial Reprints Department, Elsevier Inc., 360 Park Avenue South, New York, New York 10010-1710. Tel.: 212-633-3874; Fax: 212-633-3820; E-mail: reprints@elsevier.com.

Urologic Clinics of North America is covered in MEDLINE/PubMed (*Index Medicus*), *Excerpta Medica, Current Contents/Clinical Medicine, Science Citation Index,* and *ISI/BIOMED.*

Contributors

EDITOR-IN-CHIEF

KEVIN R. LOUGHLIN, MD, MBA
Emeritus Professor of Surgery (Urology),
Harvard Medical School, Visiting Scientist,
Vascular Biology Research Program at Boston
Children's Hospital, Boston, Massachusetts,
USA

EDITOR

TRACY M. DOWNS, MD, FACS
Professor, Department of Urology, University
of Virginia, Senior Associate Dean, Diversity,
Equity, and Inclusion, University of Virginia
School of Medicine, Chief Diversity and
Community Engagement Officer, University of
Virginia Health System, Charlottesville,
Virginia, USA

AUTHORS

OLUTIWA AKINSOLA, MD, MS
Urology Resident, Department of Urology,
Vanderbilt University Medical Center,
Nashville, Tennessee, USA

SOHRAB ARORA, MD, MS, MCh
Vattikuti Urology Institute, Henry Ford Health,
Detroit, Michigan, USA

HUMPHREY O. ATIEMO, MD
Vattikuti Urology Institute, Henry Ford Health,
Detroit, Michigan, USA

RAM BASAK, PhD
Department of Urology, School of Medicine,
The University of North Carolina at Chapel Hill,
Chapel Hill, North Carolina, USA

EMMA C. BETHEL, MD
Department of Urology, School of Medicine,
The University of North Carolina at Chapel Hill,
Chapel Hill, North Carolina, USA

KRISTY M. BORAWSKI, MD
Department of Urology, School of Medicine,
The University of North Carolina at Chapel Hill,
Chapel Hill, North Carolina, USA

CHRISTI BUTLER, MD
Assistant Professor, University of California,
San Francisco, San Francisco, California, USA

JEFFREY CARBONELLA, MD
Department of Urology, Yale School of
Medicine, New Haven, Connecticut, USA

JESSICA CLARK, MD
Department of Urology, Lewis Katz School of
Medicine, Temple University, Philadelphia,
Pennsylvania, USA

STEPHANIE DAIGNAULT-NEWTON, MS
Department of Urology, Michigan Medicine,
University of Michigan, Ann Arbor, Michigan,
USA

ALYSEN DEMZIK, MD
Department of Urology, School of Medicine,
The University of North Carolina at Chapel Hill,
Chapel Hill, North Carolina, USA

ELODI J. DIELUBANZA, MD
Brigham and Women's Hospital, Boston,
Massachusetts, USA

LAURA DOUGLASS, MD
Assistant Professor, Department of Urology,
Lewis Katz School of Medicine, Temple
University, Philadelphia, Pennsylvania,
USA

GEOLANI W. DY, MD
Associate Professor, Department of Urology,
Oregon Health and Science University,
Portland, Oregon, USA

PAULINE FILIPPOU, MD
Department of Urology, Kaiser Permanente
Northern California, Santa Clara Medical
Center, Santa Clara, California, USA

MAURICE M. GARCIA, MD, MAS
Departments of Urology and Anatomy,
University of California, San Francisco, San
Francisco, California, USA; Associate
Professor, Department of Urology, Director,
Cedars-Sinai Transgender Surgery and Health
Program, Fellowship Director, Gender
Affirming Genital Surgery and Sexual Medicine,
Cedars-Sinai Medical Center, Los Angeles, Los
Angeles, California, USA

STEPHANIE HANCHUK, MD
Department of Urology, Yale School of
Medicine, New Haven, Connecticut,
USA

FINN HENNIG, BS
Medical Student, Jacobs School of Medicine
and Biomedical Sciences, University of
Buffalo, Buffalo, New York, USA

LINDSEY A. HERREL, MD, MS
Department of Urology, Michigan Medicine,
University of Michigan, Ann Arbor, Michigan,
USA

TASHZNA JONES, MD
Department of Urology, Yale School of
Medicine, New Haven, Connecticut,
USA

MIN JUN, DO
Crane Center for Transgender Surgery,
Greenbrae, California, USA

HANNAH E. KAY, MD
Department of Urology, School of Medicine,
The University of North Carolina at Chapel Hill,
Chapel Hill, North Carolina, USA

PARIS KELLY, MS
Quinnipiac University, Hamden, Connecticut,
USA

ADAM P. KLAUSNER, MD
Professor and Endeavour Legacy Foundation
Distinguished Chair, Urology Residency
Program Director, Division of Urology,
Department of Surgery, Virginia
Commonwealth University School of Medicine,
Richmond, Virginia, USA

KATE H. KRAFT, MD
Department of Urology, Michigan Medicine,
University of Michigan, Ann Arbor, Michigan,
USA

TSZ KIN LEE, MD
British Columbia Cancer, Abbotsford, British
Columbia, Canada

KEVIN R. LOUGHLIN, MD, MBA
Professor Emeritus, Harvard Medical School,
Trustee Emeritus, American Board of Urology,
Vascular Biology Research Program, Boston
Children's Hospital, Boston, Massachusetts,
USA

SUSAN M. MACDONALD, MD
Department of Urology, Penn State Health
Milton S. Hershey Medical Center, Hershey,
Pennsylvania, USA

FENIZIA MAFFUCCI, MD
Department of Urology, Lewis Katz School of
Medicine, Temple University, Philadelphia,
Pennsylvania, USA

JOANNA M. MAINWARING, BSCHONS
Department of Anatomy, University of Otago,
Dunedin, New Zealand

RENA D. MALIK, MD
Division of Urology, University of Maryland
School of Medicine, Baltimore, Maryland,
USA

ASIA N. MATTHEW-ONABANJO, MD, PhD
Department of Urology, School of Medicine,
The University of North Carolina at Chapel Hill,
Chapel Hill, North Carolina, USA

CATHERINE S. NAM, MD
Department of Urology, Michigan Medicine,
University of Michigan, Ann Arbor, Michigan,
USA

KRISTEN R. SCARPATO, MD
Associate Professor, Urology Residency
Program Director, Department of Urology,
Vanderbilt University Medical Center,
Nashville, Tennessee, USA

R. CRAIG SINEATH, MD, MPH
Resident, Department of Urology, Oregon
Health and Science University, Portland,
Oregon, USA

ANGELA B. SMITH, MD, MS
Department of Urology, School of Medicine,
The University of North Carolina at Chapel Hill,
Chapel Hill, North Carolina, USA

JOSHUA STERLING, MD, MSc
Assistant Professor, Department of Urology,
Yale School of Medicine, New Haven,
Connecticut, USA

HUNG-JUI TAN, MD, MSHPM
Department of Urology, School of
Medicine, The University of North Carolina at
Chapel Hill, Chapel Hill, North Carolina,
USA

RANDY VINCE, MD
Assistant Professor and Director of Minority
Men's Health, Case Western Reserve
University, University Hospital Urology
Institute, Cleveland, Ohio, USA

DAVIS VIPRAKASIT, MD
Department of Urology, School of Medicine,
The University of North Carolina at Chapel Hill,
Chapel Hill, North Carolina, USA

ERIC M. WALLEN, MD
Department of Urology, School of Medicine,
The University of North Carolina at Chapel Hill,
Chapel Hill, North Carolina, USA

RICHARD J. WASSERSUG, PhD
Department of Cellular and Physiological
Sciences, University of British Columbia,
Vancouver, Canada

ERIK WIBOWO, PhD
Department of Anatomy, University of Otago,
Dunedin, New Zealand

Contents

Vivien Thomas was born into humble beginnings in Iberia, Louisiana in 1910. The circumstances of that era prevented him from achieving his goal of attending medical school. He became a surgical research technician at Vanderbilt Medical School. While at Vanderbilt, he began working under Alfred Blalock, one of the famous surgeons of that era. When Blalock left Vanderbilt, he asked Thomas to come with him. At Hopkins, the surgical procedure known as the Blalock-Taussig Shunt was developed to treat a serious congenital heart defect known as Tetralogy of Fallot. Vivien Thomas was instrumental in the development of that procedure.

Workforce and Diversity

Analysis of the urology match statistics provides a window into the future of the urology workforce. Match statistics from 2019 to 2023 were analyzed to determine whether the efforts to promote diversity in 2020 have been impactful. The popularity in the field of urology among all racial/ethnic groups peaked interest in application in 2022. However despite an increase in URIM applicants over the last 5 years, 2023 URM applicants have 1/3 the odds of matching into urology as white applicants.

Multiple estimates have approximated a urologist shortage per capita of around 30% by 2030. In the context of the impending urologic workforce shortage, it is critical to have a nuanced understanding of the degree of workforce shortage in comparison with the US population to mitigate the negative downstream effects in the future. In continued growth and stagnant growth projection models, we found that female urologists make up a significant proportion of the workforce growth over the next four decades. This projection highlights the need for purposeful recruitment, structural changes, and advocacy among urology leadership to support and retain female urologists.

examined the item content and documentation of validation. These scales predominantly focus on general sexual function and erection. They lack questions on behaviors relevant to men-who-have-sex-with-men (MSM), such as anal sex, masturbation, or sexual activities outside of committed relationships. Additionally, the validation samples rarely mention inclusion of MSM, revealing a clear gap in the clinical evaluation tools available for MSM, who are experiencing sexual dysfunction from prostate cancer treatment side effects.

UROLOGIC CLINICS OF NORTH AMERICA

SERIES OF RELATED INTEREST
Surgical Clinics of North America
https://www.surgical.theclinics.com/

Foreword
Diversity in Urology: The Time Is Now

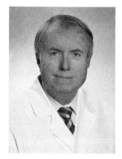

Kevin R. Loughlin, MD, MBA,
Editor-in-Chief

This issue of *Urologic Clinics*, Diversity in Urology, is long overdue. It gives me great pleasure as editor-in-chief to have enlisted Tracy Downs, MD and other experts, who have contributed to this issue to produce a truly landmark volume on this topic.

Unfortunately, the struggle for diversity and equality continues throughout our society and in urologic practice as well.[1] The 2021 American Urological Association (AUA) Census reported the racial breakdown of 13,790 urologic practitioners was white 83.3%, Asian 12.8%, black or African American 2.4%, and other races, including multiple races, 1.4%.

The 2021 census did not define Hispanic as race, but as an ethnicity. Using that categorization, the census reported 4.4% of practitioners as Hispanic and 95.6% as non-Hispanic.[2] The 2021 AUA Census also reports that only 10.9% of practicing urologists as female.[3]

Sarah Psutka, a urologic oncologist and Associate Professor of Urology at the University of Washington, is leading an initiative to increase female leadership in urology. She makes the compelling recommendation, "It is incredibly important to increase opportunities among women as well as other underrepresented groups. Facilitating diversity and

equity in both representation within the ranks of leadership is critical."[2]

In addition to the need for greater attention to be paid to racial and gender diversity in urology, there is also a need for greater representation in the LGBTQ community. Sineath and colleagues[4] have recently published a report outlining how to better serve this constituency.

The goal to achieve diversity in urology needs to start during medical school, if not earlier.[5] It is important that our leadership organizations, like the AUA and the American Board of Urology (ABU), take steps to address the problem. In December 2020, the AUA announced the formation of its Diversity and Inclusion Task Force, chaired by Tracy Downs and co-chaired by Simone Thavaseelan.[6] Similarly, the ABU has published an important document, "The American Board of Urology: In Pursuit of Diversity, Equity and Inclusion," which outlines tangible methods to build a foundation of diversity, quality, and inclusion within the Board of Urology and its certifying processes.[7]

Let me close my preface to this important issue by recalling the words of two famous, but diverse historical figures: Winston Churchill and Mahatma Gandhi. Churchill said, "Diversity is the one true

Urol Clin N Am 50 (2023) xi–xii
https://doi.org/10.1016/j.ucl.2023.06.018
0094-0143/23/© 2023 Published by Elsevier Inc.

thing we all have in common…. **Celebrate it every day.**" Gandhi said, **"Our ability to reach unity in diversity will be the beauty and the test of our civilization."** The future of urology will go as far as our diversity takes us.

Kevin R. Loughlin, MD, MBA
Visiting Scientist
Vascular Biology Research Program at
Boston Children's Hospital
300 Longwood Avenue
Boston, MA 02115, USA

E-mail address:
kloughlin@partners.org

REFERENCES

1. Loughlin KR. Diversity in urology: if not now, when? Can J Urol 2022;29(4):11198–9.

2. Available at: Healthecareers.com/career-resources/friends-and-data/diversity-among-urologists. Accessed April 14, 2023.

3. Makarov DV, Penson DF. The state of the urology workforce and practice in the United States, AUA Census, 2021. Available at: https://www.auanet.org. Accessed April 12, 2023.

4. Sineath RC, Sparks SS, Griebling TL. LGBT+ representation in urology. AUA News 2021;26(4):1–2.

5. Slaughenhoupt FB, Ogunyemi O, Giannopoulos M, et al. An update on the current status of medical school education in the United States. Urology 2014;84:743–7.

6. Downs TM, Moses K. Diversity in urology: progress made, but there is more work to be done. Urology Times 9/15/22. Available at: urologytimes.com/view/diversity-in-urology-progress-made-but-there-is-more-work-to-be-done. Accessed April 13, 2023.

7. Husmann DA, Terris MK, Lee CT, et al. The American Board of Urology: in pursuit of diversity, equity and inclusion. Urol Pract 2021;8(5):583–8.

Preface

Hold Fast and Stay True: Unmasking Our Past and Affirming Diversity and Inclusive Excellence as We Advance the Field of Urology

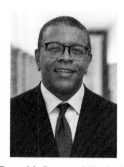

Tracy M. Downs, MD, FACS
Editor

We are concerned about the constant use of federal funds to support this most notorious expression of segregation. Of all the forms of inequality, injustice in health is the most shocking and the most inhuman because it often results in physical death.
—Reverend Dr Martin Luther King Jr, March 25, 1966 (Press Conference–Chicago at the Second Convention of the Medical Committee for Human Rights [MCHR])

Diversity, Equity, and Inclusion (DEI) work is not new as some would want you to believe. In fact, in the United States, it has its roots in the 1960s Civil Rights Movement and has grown to include gender, sexual orientation, religion, country of origin, and other identities. The focus in the 1960s and into the mid-1970s was on tolerance, meaning the acceptance of integration of workplaces, schools, and communities. Later in the mid-1970s and into the 1990s, the focus was on multiculturalism and being aware of the achievements of various racial and ethnic minorities. In our contemporary moment, DEI work is linked to our strategic vision(s) as health care organizations to provide patient-centered care to all of our patients and diverse communities, through intentional initiatives to (a) improve workforce diversity, (b) train culturally responsive and competent health care providers for a global society, (c) authenticate partnerships with local leaders/community organizations to promote health, and (d) socially respond to educational curriculums/teaching that leads to improved patient outcomes, a reduction in biased health care, and discoveries in research that benefit all human beings from a multitude of diverse backgrounds.

As a self-described collector of quotes, one quote that I was exposed to during my urologic residency training years, by one of my professors that really aligns with the core essence of Inclusion, is the quote "All of us are smarter than one of us" by Kevin R. Loughlin, MD.

This issue of *Urologic Clinics* provides a tremendous overview of the scope of DEI across the breadth of our specialty. I am grateful to the authors, all of whom are well-recognized global experts in their respective fields of interest.

Tracy M. Downs, MD, FACS
Department of Urology
University of Virginia School of Medicine
UVA Health System
1415 Lee Street
Charlottesville, VA 22908-0813, USA

E-mail address:
tracymdowns@virginia.edu

Urol Clin N Am 50 (2023) xiii
https://doi.org/10.1016/j.ucl.2023.06.019
0094-0143/23/© 2023 Published by Elsevier Inc.

Vivien Thomas
His Legacy and Lessons

Kevin R. Loughlin, MD, MBA*

KEYWORDS

- Surgical research • Diversity • Equity • Inclusion

KEY POINTS

- Vivien Thomas was a surgical research technician at Johns Hopkins who was instrumental in developing the Blalock-Taussig repair of the Tetralogy of Fallot.
- As an African American without a medical degree, it was many years before he received the recognition that he deserved.
- He applied not only his surgical skill but also his intellect and creativity to the development of the surgical repair of this serious congenital heart defect.
- His life and career are reminders that the struggle for diversity, equity, and inclusion continues in the medical profession to this day.

HUMBLE BEGINNINGS

He was born in rural Louisiana in 1910, the grandson of a slave and the son of a carpenter. He learned carpentry from his father, but from an early age his dream was to become a doctor. In that era, he realized that few African Americans went on to become physicians, but he dreamed his dream nonetheless.

His family moved to Nashville, Tennessee and he did not let go of his dream.

He saved money from carpentry jobs and planned to enroll at Tennessee A & I State College. Then the depression came; his savings were wiped out, and his dreams were shattered.[1]

THE VANDERBILT YEARS

However, he was undeterred and got a job at Vanderbilt Medical School. He was hired by a young surgeon, Alfred Blalock, to work in the surgical research laboratory. In an era when institutional racism was the norm, he was classified and paid as a "janitor" despite the fact that he was doing the work of a postdoctoral researcher in Blalock's laboratory.

Working in Blalock's laboratory, Vivien Thomas soon learned how much he loved surgery.

Blalock's early interest was in the physiology of shock. Many investigators of the time erroneously thought shock was due to "toxins" and other mediators of hypotension. Blalock, with Thomas' help, gained medical notoriety in establishing that shock was fundamentally caused by fluid loss and decreased circulatory blood volume. Blalock's reputation, not Thomas', grew, and as a result, Blalock was recruited back to Johns Hopkins, where he had gone to medical school, as chief of surgery, one of the most prestigious positions in the medical profession.

TETRALOGY OF FALLOT

Upon arrival at Johns Hopkins, Blalock found the surgical research laboratories badly in need of expansion and renovation. He essentially delegated these tasks to Thomas. Thomas enthusiastically took this on and became intimately involved with animal surgery in the research laboratory. It became readily apparent to all who observed that Thomas had a gift for surgery. He quickly became a mentor to the surgical residents at Hopkins. A testimony to the regard in which Thomas was held by the surgical residents is demonstrated by a story by Dr Alex Haller, who

Harvard Medical School
* Vascular Biology Laboratory, Boston Children's Hospital, Longwood Avenue, Boston, MA 02115.
E-mail address: kloughlin@partners.org

Urol Clin N Am 50 (2023) 491–493
https://doi.org/10.1016/j.ucl.2023.06.008

later would become chief of pediatric surgery at Hopkins.

Haller was at the National Institutes of Health following his surgical training and was performing animal surgery alone, except for a technician, Mr Alfred Casper. They encountered some massive bleeding, which Haller was able to control. Afterward, Casper complimented Haller on the manner in which he controlled the bleeding. Haller, feeling proud of himself, replied, "Well, I was trained by Dr Blalock." A few weeks later, operating together again on an animal, Haller and Casper encountered another episode of profuse bleeding, and Casper helped Haller get out of trouble. Haller turned to Casper and thanked him and told him how impressed he was with his surgical skills. Casper replied,"Well, I trained with Vivien."[2]

Soon after Blalock arrived at Hopkins, he was introduced to Helen Taussig, the Chief of Pediatric Cardiology. Taussig was challenged by and interested in infants with the "blue baby" syndrome. The underlying cardiac defect in these children was what was known as the Tetralogy of Fallot. The Tetralogy of Fallot consisted of (1) ventricular septal defect; (2) an overriding aorta; (3) pulmonary stenosis; and (4) right ventricular hypertrophy.[3] This constellation of congenital defects causes too little blood to reach the lungs. This low oxygen (blue) blood then circulates to the rest of the body with insufficient oxygen reaching the body tissues.[4]

Taussig was hoping that some surgeon could "reconnect the pipes" to permit more oxygenated blood to reach the body.[5] In 1943, she had approached the renowned Robert Gross of Boston Children's Hospital about the possibility of surgical repair without success.[6] Taussig continued to be curious about whether there could be a surgical solution for the Tetralogy of Fallot. She and Blalock began to have further discussions regarding the potential of surgical repair.

Taussig had observed that children with a cyanotic heart defect and a patent ductus arteriosus (PDA) seemed to live longer than those without a PDA.[6] This suggested to her that a shunt that mimicked the function of a PDA might solve the problem of poor oxygenation by getting more blood to the lungs. She viewed it "as a plumber changes pipes around."[6]

Fortuitously, Blalock and Thomas, while at Vanderbilt, had worked on a subclavian artery to pulmonary artery shunt for a different purpose. They therefore had some familiarity with a potential solution. They took the problem to the surgical research laboratory at Hopkins, where Thomas performed a subclavian to pulmonary artery anastomosis on 200 dogs. After they both became convinced of the reliability of the surgery, they, along with Taussig, decided to proceed on a child.

On November 29, 1943, they tried the procedure on an 18-month-old infant named Eileen Saxon.[5] Blalock performed the surgery, and Thomas, although not allowed to scrub, was by his side. As no specific instruments for cardiac surgery then existed, Thomas adapted instruments from the laboratory for Blalock to use. Thomas, reportedly, coached Blalock, step by step, through the procedure.[5] This first case was not completely successful but did prolong the girl's life for several months. This case and 2 subsequent cases were published as a series in the May 1945 issue of the *Journal of the American Medical Association*.[5] Blalock and Taussig were included as authors; Thomas was not.[5]

The original Blalock-Taussig shunt has been modified since its original description, but the basic concept of shunting blood to the lungs to increase oxygenation has remained unchanged.

THE RACIAL ENVIRONMENT AT HOPKINS

Blalock and Taussig gained worldwide notoriety for their operation. Despite his contributions, Thomas remained in obscurity. In the 1940s, Baltimore was very much a southern city with rigid segregation, and Johns Hopkins remained a very southern school. Despite Thomas' role as Chief of the Surgical Research Laboratory, the only other African American employees at Hopkins at that time were janitors.[5] When Thomas needed to walk to Blalock's office in the hospital, he would remove his white coat and change into his city clothes. Although his contributions to the surgery department were critical, he was not well paid. To earn extra income, he would sometimes work as a bartender at Blalock's parties and serve drinks to the surgical residents who he had been training earlier in the day.

LIKE SOMETHING THE LORD MADE

Despite some interpersonal tensions, Blalock and Thomas continued to work together. In 1946, they began to work on the surgical correction of a congenital abnormality known as Transposition of the Great Vessels. Blalock visited Thomas in the research laboratory, and upon examining an anastomosis that Thomas had performed, commented, "Vivien, this looks like something the Lord made." This phrase would later serve as the title of an article about the life of Vivien Thomas and an HBO movie.[7]

Thomas' technical skills became legendary. Notable surgeons, such as Denton Cooley,

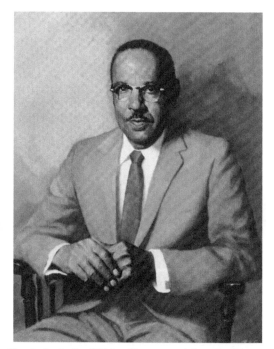

Fig. 1. Portrait of Vivien Thomas at Johns Hopkins.

Rowena Spencer, Alex Haller, and Frank Spencer, credited Thomas with some of the superb surgical training they received. Cooley commented, "There wasn't a false move, not a wasted motion, when he operated."[7]

RECOGNITION DELAYED, BUT NOT DENIED

Vivien Thomas served at Johns Hopkins Medical School for 37 years.

Because of the enormous regard in which he was held throughout the surgical department, the recognition that he so richly deserved began to accrue over time. The Blalock-Thomas shunt began to be known as the Blalock-Thomas-Taussig shunt. In 1968, surgeons that Thomas had helped train commissioned a portrait of him that was hung next to Blalock's in the lobby of the Alfred Blalock Clinical Sciences Building **(Fig. 1)**.[5]

In 1976, Johns Hopkins University awarded Thomas an honorary degree.

Because of certain rubrics, he received an Honorary Doctor of Laws, rather than a medical doctorate, but the university allowed him to be addressed as "doctor."

Finally, he was also appointed to the faculty of the School of Medicine as Instructor of Surgery.

ENDURING LEGACY—LESSONS LEARNED

It is easy to discount the injustices suffered by Vivien Thomas to a different era, but that would be naive. Perhaps just as pervasive as racism is the continued arrogation by senior clinicians and department Chairs of their junior colleagues' work.

We must not forget that the medical profession is a reflection of the society in which we work. In the same fashion that our society struggles to move forward and correct prior inequities, so must our profession. Vivien Thomas' contributions go far beyond the surgical techniques he pioneered and the surgeons he helped train. His legacy of humility, determination, and hard work is a precious inheritance for all of us in the medical profession. Thank you, Doctor Thomas.

CLINICS CARE POINTS

- Research recognition is often unfair.
- Senior physicians are responsible for fairness and academic integrity in their publications.

REFERENCES

1. The Unlikely Legacy of Vivien Thomas. Medical Bag.https:U www.medicalbag.com/home/specia lities/physician-assistants/the- unlikely-legacy-of-vivien-thomas .Accessed 9/16/2019.
2. Kennedy DM. In search of Vivien Thomas. Texas Heart Journal 2005;32(4):477–8.
3. Tetralogy of Fallot (TOF). Children's Hospital of Philadelphia. https:www.chop.edu/conditions-diseases/tetralogy-fallot. Accessed 12/16/2019.
4. Tetralogy of Fallot(TOF) Reviewed by Gina Baffa MD. https:U kidshealth.org/en/parents/tetralogy-of-fallot.html. Accessed 12/16/2019.
5. Wikipedia. Vivien Thomas. https://en.wikipedia.org/wikiN i vien Thomas. Accessed 9/6/2019.
6. Wikipedia. Blalock-Taussig shunt. https://en.wikipedia.org/Blalock-Taussig shunt. 12/16/2019.
7. McCabe K. Like something the Lord made. Washington, DC: Washingtonian magazine; 1989.

Workforce and Diversity

Diversity in Urology, Are We Moving in the Right Direction?
Analysis of American Urologic Association Urology Residency Match Statistics 2019–2023

Elodi J. Dielubanza, MD[a], Sohrab Arora, MD, MS, MCh[b], Humphrey O. Atiemo, MD[b],*

KEYWORDS

- Diversity • Disparity • Urology match • Workforce

KEY POINTS

- Since 2020, there has been an increase in underrepresented in medicine (URM) applications for urology residency.
- The URM match rate is statistically unchanged over the last 5 years and continues to be lower than white applicants.
- The match rate of Black and Hispanic/Latino applicants seem to be inversely proportional.
- Progress is slow, and the full impact of the diversity equity, and inclusion efforts in urology have not been realized.

INTRODUCTION

Racial disparities within the US health system[1] impact access to care, representation in clinical trials,[2] morbidity, and mortality.[3,4] Diversifying the medical workforce has been a key focus in beginning to address these disparities. The current state of progress toward improved diversity, equity, and inclusion (DEI) in the urology workforce is not well documented and there is limited research on the subject. However, it is generally accepted that urology workforce diversity does not reflect that of the community at large.[5] Urologists have traditionally been predominantly male and nonHispanic White. Black/African American, Hispanic/Latino, Native American, and Asian Pacific Islander/Native Alaskan groups comprise one-third of the US population, yet they constitute <15% of the urology workforce. Whereas Asian Americans make up 6% of the US population, they comprise 12.8% of urologists. Women represent 50.5% of the US population, but only 10.9% of urologists.[6] According to 2021 American Urological Association (AUA) census data, only 2.4% of practicing urologists in the United States are Black or African American, and 4.4% are Hispanic or Latino.

Note: race/ethnicity denotes that both race and ethnicity were combined in this analysis, but that race and ethnicity are distinctly different and not synonymous.

a Brigham and Women's Hospital, 45 Francis Street, Boston, MA 02115, USA; b Vattikuti Urology Institute Henry Ford Health, 2799 West Grand Boulevard, K9, Detroit, MI 48202, USA

* Corresponding author.

E-mail address: hatiemo1@hfhs.org

Urol Clin N Am 50 (2023) 495–500

https://doi.org/10.1016/j.ucl.2023.06.010

The events of 2020 were an important social inflection point. The devastation of the SARS-COVID-19 pandemic highlighted the disparate impact of disease on racial and ethnic minorities regarding morbidity and mortality.[7] The murder of Mr. George Floyd was also a catalyst for a national conversation about racism and a re-examination of the progress of DEI in many sectors including education and health care. The urologic community was not immune to the social upheaval of 2020. In recent years, there has been greater awareness of the racial disparities in the urological workforce with several training programs promoting DEI initiatives to improve the matriculation of URM urologists in the profession. One of the most significant aspects of DEI initiatives is to measure the impact of their effect. Analysis of urology match statistics allows for a unique measurement of diversity by assessing the racial and ethnic diversity of future urological physicians and leaders. The primary aim of this study is to measure the diversity of applicants in the urology residency match and the success of URM applicants in the match before and after the year 2020.

METHODS

The AUA match data were queried from 2019 to 2023. Subjects were assessed for match results and self-reported race and ethnicity. Applicants were stratified by their self-reported racial and ethnic diversity. Racial and ethnic groups were classified as White, Asian, Hispanic/Latino, African American, Native American, and Pacific Islander. Underrepresented in medicine (URM) was defined as African American, Hispanic/Latino and Native American, and Pacific Islander. The total number of applicants per year, URM applicants per year, and match rates per year for each racial/ethnic group were assessed. Chi-squared analysis was used to assess the match rate of each racial/ethnic group by year and the match rate between racial/ethnic groups. A proportional test was applied for the racial/ethnic distribution of those who matched versus year, and those who applied versus year. Statistical analysis of the Native American/Pacific Islander group was not performed due to the single-digit number of applicants. Applicants with unknown race and ethnicity were not included in the analysis. Statistical significance was set at a P value of less than 0.05. Of note, race/ethnicity applicant and match statistics before 2019 could not be analyzed as the AUA did not collect these data until 2019.

RESULTS

From 2019 to 2023 there was a statistically significant annual increase in the number of urology residency applicants (**Table 1**). The number of applications peaked in 2022 with a 42% increase from 389 applications in 2019 to 555 applicants in 2022, followed by a nonsignificant decrease in the number of applicants in 2023. The number of urology residency positions also increased during this period from 330 to 385. Applicants from URM groups increased over the study period from 49 (13%) in 2019 to 110 (22%) in 2023. This increase was driven largely by a nearly three-fold increase in the Hispanic/Latino applicants (26 in 2019 to 71 in 2023). Black applicants increased as well from 24 to 37 applications (**Table 2**). Compared with 2019, the 2023 data demonstrated a 10% decrease in the number of white applicants and a 10% increase in URM applicants (**Table 3**). The number of white applicants exceeded the number of Asian and URM applicants throughout the study period. There was minimal change in the percentage of Black and Asian applicants over the 5 year period, representing 8% and 24%, respectively. Interestingly, there was a decrease in the number of applicants who identified as "Other" from 11% to 4% (**Fig. 1**).

There was a statically significant decrease in the overall match rate that occurred over the 5 year

	2019		2020		2021		2022		2023		
RACE/URM	**N**	**%**	**N**	**%**	**N**	**%**	**N**	**%**	**N**	**%**	**P-value**
White	206	53	212	48	233	49	283	51	275	54	<.001
URM	49	13	80	18	103	21	110	20	110	22	
Asian	90	23	103	23	104	22	116	21	102	20	
Other	44	11	46	10	40	8	46	8	20	4	
Total	389		441		480		555		507		
Available Residency Position	330		353		357		365		385		

Table 1
Urology applicants/year and available residency position

Table 2
2019–2023 racial distribution of applicants

RACE/URM	2019		2023		
	N	%	N	%	P-value
White	206	60	275	57	0.003
Black	24	7	37	8	
Asian	90	26	102	21	
Hispanic, Latino	23	7	71	15	
Total	343		485		

study period (**Fig. 2**). The lowest match rate was 66% in 2022 that coincided with the peak number of applications. The URM match rate also declined from 80% in 2019 to 61% in 2023, though this was not statistically significant.

The highest URM match rate occurred in 2019 and 2020, 39 of 49 (79.5%) and 63 of 80 (78.7%), representing 13% and 18% of all matched applicants, in those years, respectively. Thereafter, the match rate for URM applicants has remained at approximately 60%, maintaining ~18% of matched positions overall (**Fig. 3**). Interestingly, when examining the trend among racial/ethnic subgroups there is a differential impact regarding the trend in declining match rate. There was an inverse relationship between match success in Black and Hispanic/Latino applicants. From 2019 to 2022, there was a continuous decline in the match rate of Hispanic/Latino applicants from 87% to 44%, whereas Black applicants had a modest increase in the match rate from 71% to 73% during the same period. The Black applicant match rate was highest in 2020 at 82%. The 2023 match saw an 18% increase in the Hispanic/Latino match with a 14% decrease in the Black match rate (**Fig. 4**).

American Indian/Alaska Native represent the fewest number of applicants in the Urology Match. In 2019 only 2 individuals from this ethnic group applied for the match. The peak number of American Indian/Alaska Native applicants was 5 in 2021

Table 3
White vs underrepresented in medicine applicants

RACE/URM	2019		2023		
	N	%	N	%	P-value
White	206	81	275	71	0.007
URM	49	19	110	29	
Total	255		385		

and 2022 and there were no applicants from this group in 2020. The match rate was 64% over the 5 year period (**Fig. 5**, **Table 4**).

DISCUSSION

The disparity in representation in the Urology workforce has been a topic of great interest in recent years. Racial and ethnic diversity in training programs will position the future workforce to better address social determinants of health and the unique needs of different communities.[8,9] A representative workforce not only provides culturally sensitive care that can improve physician–patient relationships, but also has been shown to improve patient outcomes.[10] Although equity and inclusion are more complex concepts requiring a multifaceted approach, diversity is a more measurable statistic that can potentially improve the care gap. Fortunately, there has been a drive to increase awareness of this issue over the last several years leading to the AUA announcement of instituting a formal diversity and inclusion committee in 2022.

The 2021 AUA census determined that the number of practicing urologists with White ethnicity is 83.3%, Hispanic ethnicity 4.4%, and African American/Black ethnicity 2.4%.[6] This contrasts with the 2022 United States Census data which demonstrate that Hispanic/Latino and African American/Black individuals make up 18.9% and 13.6% of the US population, respectively, whereas White Americans make up 75.8% of the population.[11] To address this gap, many training programs have promoted DEI initiatives.[12–14] However, the effects of DEI efforts on the workforce will take many years to realize. A review of the Urology match data provides a window into the progress toward diversity and an opportunity to identify areas for improvement. During the study period, there was a 30% increase in the number of urology applicants and only a 14% increase in Urology positions, resulting in historically low match rates. Nevertheless, White and Asian applicants retained a consistent proportion of total applications and a similar proportion of successful applications. Conversely, the proportion of matched Black candidates was progressively lower than the proportion of Black applicants. In 2019, Black students comprised 8.7% of applicants and matched at a rate of 8.8%. In comparison, 2021 demonstrated a reduction in the number of Black applicants and match rate of 6.3% and 5.3% respectively. The same pattern was observed for Hispanic applicants. These data suggest disparities in the acceptance rate for Black and Hispanic candidates. This is likely multifactorial. Identifying the actionable causes of these

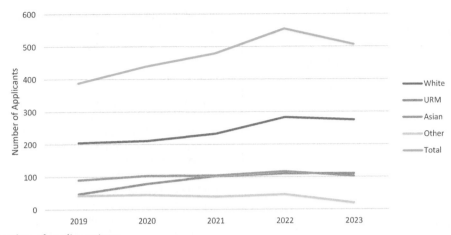

Fig. 1. Number of applicants/year.

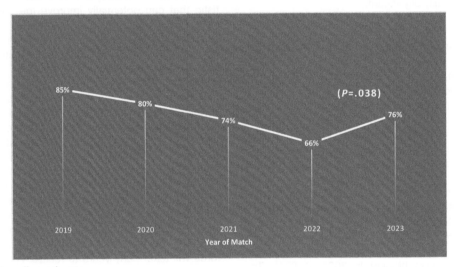

Fig. 2. Overall match rate.

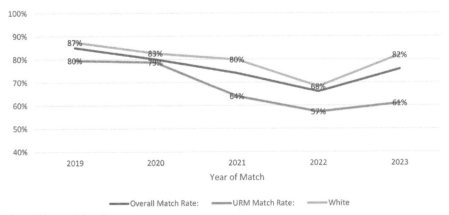

Fig. 3. URM vs white match rate.

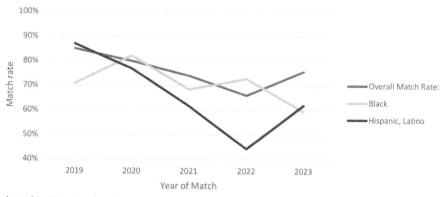

Fig. 4. Black and Latino match rate.

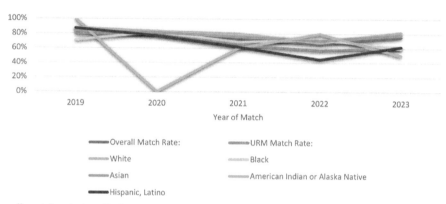

Fig. 5. Overall match rate by ethnic group.

disparities and taking appropriate actions to address them is key to enriching the workforce. Authors at one institution used a 3 prong approach to URM recruitment with targeted outreach to candidates, funding support for visiting clerkship, holistic review of applications, and targeted outreach to candidates. With this approach, the number of URM interviewees significantly increased from 6.1% in 2015 to its peak, 40%, in 2020 with an increase in the complement of URM residents from 0% in 2015 to 35% in 2022.[15–17]

Consistent efforts over the next few decades will be needed to fully actualize the DEI goals of the urology profession.

Although the DEI initiative in urology does not have the full force of federal law like Title IX of the Education Amendments of 1972, lessons can be learned from the 50 years of its implementation. Before Title IX 1 in 27 girls played sports and today 2 in 5 girls play sports.[18] In 1970 only 9% of medical school enrollment was composed of women and in 2023 women comprised about 53% of medical school enrollment.[19] Diversity in urology residency training and subsequent workforce will take time. The updated match statistics in this current study demonstrate that urology is moving in the right direction; however, the needle moves slowly, and although progress is slow, it is still in progress.

DISCLOSURE

The authors have no financial disclosure or declarations of Interest to report.

Table 4 Applicant by ethnicity					
Applicant by Ethnicity	**2019**	**2020**	**2021**	**2022**	**2023**
White	206	212	233	283	275
Black	24	28	38	44	37
Asian	90	103	104	116	102
American Indian or Alaska Native	2	0	5	5	2
Hispanic, Latino	23	52	60	61	71
Undisclosed Ethnicity	34	35	30	31	11
Other	10	11	10	15	9

REFERENCES

1. Williams DR, Rucker TD. Understanding and addressing racial disparities in health care. Health Care Financ Rev 2000;21(4):75–90. PMID: 11481746; PMCID: PMC4194634.
2. Alsan M, Wanamaker M. Tuskegee and the health of black men. Q J Econ 2018;133(1):407.
3. Benjamins MR, Silva A, Saiyed NS, et al. Comparison of all-cause mortality rates and inequities between black and white populations across the 30 most populous US cities. JAMA Netw Open 2021; 4(1):e2032086.
4. Mokdad AH, Dwyer-Lindgren L, Fitzmaurice C, et al. Trends and patterns of disparities in cancer mortality among US Counties, 1980-2014. JAMA, J Am Med Assoc 2017;317(4):388–406.
5. Simons ECG, Arevalo A, Washington SL, et al. Trends in the racial and ethnic diversity in the US urology workforce. Urology 2022;162:9–19.
6. The State of the Urology Workforce and Practice in the United States: AUA CENSUS 2021 Census Results - American Urological Association. Available at: https://www.auanet.org/research-and-data/aua-census/census-results. Accessed January 16, 2023.
7. Schumm LP, Giurcanu MC, Locey KJ, et al. Racial and ethnic disparities in the observed COVID-19 case fatality rate among the U.S. population. Ann Epidemiol 2022;74:118–24.
8. Komaromy M, Grumbach K, Drake M, et al. The role of black and Hispanic physicians in providing health care for underserved populations. N Engl J Med 1996;334(20):1305–10.
9. Coates E, Moore C, Watson A, et al. "It's important to work with people that look like me": black patients' preferences for patient-provider race concordance. J Racial Ethn Heal Disparities 2022. https://doi.org/10.1007/S40615-022-01435-Y.
10. Tucker CM, Marsiske M, Rice KG, et al. Patient-centered culturally sensitive health care: model testing and refinement. Health Psychol 2011;30(3):342.
11. United States Census Bureau 2022: Quick Facts: Available at: https://www.census.gov/quickfacts/fact/table/US/IPE120221. Accessed January 16, 2023.
12. Azari S, Goddard B, Mehta A. How well do urology residency program webpages recruit underrepresented minorities? Can J Urol 2023;29(3):11150–3. MEDLINE is the source for the citation and abstract for this record.
13. Persad-Paisley EM, Kazal FH, Shamshad A, et al. Applying representation quotient methodology to racial, ethnic, and gender trends of applicants and matriculants to urology residency programs from 2010-2018. Urology 2023;172:25–32. Epub 2022 Nov 17. PMID: 36402268.
14. Wallace NO, Pittman AB, Wilson SN. The R frank jones urology interest group: an intentional and strategic pipeline program to increase diversity in urology. Urology 2022;162:27–32. Epub 2021 Oct 16. PMID: 34666122.
15. Williams C, Familusi O, Kovell RC, et al. Representation matters: one urology residency program's approach to increasing workforce diversity. Urology 2023;174:28–34. Epub 2022 Dec 28. PMID: 36586426.
16. Shantharam G, Tran TY, McGee H, et al. Examining trends in underrepresented minorities in urology residency. Urology 2019;127:36–41.
17. Santosa KB, Priest CR, Oliver JD, et al. Influence of faculty diversity on resident diversity across surgical subspecialties. Am J Surg 2022;224(1 Pt B):273–81.
18. Available at: https://news.harvard.edu/gazette/story/2022/06/how-title-ix-transformed-colleges-universities-over-past-50-years/Accessed 4 10, 2023.
19. Applicants, Matriculants, and Enrollment to U.S. Medical Schools by Gender: AAMC Applicant Matriculant Data File and AAMC Student Records System as of 10/31/2022. Available at: https://www.aamc.org/data-reports/students-residents/data/2022-facts-applicants-and-matriculants-data. Accessed April 10, 2023.

The Future is Female
Urology Workforce Projection from 2020 to 2057

Catherine S. Nam, MD*, Stephanie Daignault-Newton, MS,
Kate H. Kraft, MD, Lindsey A. Herrel, MD, MS

KEYWORDS

- Female • Projection • Urology • Workforce

KEY POINTS

- Median age range of the female urology workforce is significantly younger than the male cohort, which contributes to the decline in the median age range of overall urology workforce in the coming decades.
- The total number of practicing urologists per capita will decrease in the coming decade, even with continued growth of the resident complement across urology training programs, and will not recover to baseline until 2042.
- There will be an exaggerated and prolonged shortage of total urologists per ≥65 years populations in both models of our projections.
- Female urologists per capita will continue to increase in the context of decreasing urologists per capita in continued growth and stagnant growth models.
- Collectively, these projections highlight the severity of the impending shortage of urologists and importance of structural change and advocacy to maximize the available urologic workforce.

INTRODUCTION

Multiple estimates have approximated a urologist shortage per capita of around 30% by 2030.[1,2] This shortage is multifactorial. First, the Balanced Budget Act of 1997, which limits funding for residency training and caps the number of government subsidized residency positions for all medical subspecialties. Second, practicing urologists are the second oldest surgical subspecialists, with a median age of 55 years.[3] Third, the demand for urologists is expected to increase with the impending "silver tsunami," where by 2030, one in five Americans will be 65 years or older, and the Medicare population is known to disproportionately use urologic services three-times greater than the general population.[4]

Therefore, there have been projections that even if we were to maintain the current urologists per capita, there will be a shortage of urologists by 46% by 2035.[4] The importance and severity of impending urologic workforce shortage has been recognized by American Urological Association (AUA) as a federal advocacy priority with only 38% of all US counties currently with practicing urologists, recent declines in urologists per capita, and older median age of urologists. This has significant downstream consequences on access to care, delays for surgical evaluation, longer travel time for rural patients to access surgical care, and heightened pressure on practicing urologists to meet the increased demands, leading to physician burnout.[3]

Note: race/ethnicity denotes that race and ethnicity were combined in this analysis, but that race and ethnicity are distinctly different and not synonymous.
Department of Urology, Michigan Medicine University of Michigan, Ann Arbor, MI, USA
* Corresponding author. Department of Urology, University of Michigan, 1500 East Medical Center Drive, SPC 5330, Ann Arbor, MI 48105-5330.
E-mail address: namcs@med.umich.edu

Urol Clin N Am 50 (2023) 501–513
https://doi.org/10.1016/j.ucl.2023.06.011

The gender composition of the urology workforce has changed dramatically over the past few decades. Initial female representation in urology was low with only 0.9% of urology residents being women in 1978 and 22 practicing female urologists in 1985.[5,6] Although it continues to be male dominated, less so only to orthopedic surgery and neurosurgery, urology has experienced an 11-fold increase in female representation from 1978 to 2013, the largest growth among all specialties.[5] Currently, 10.9% of practicing urologists are female, and 30.9% of urology residents are female.[7,8]

Although there have been multiple projection studies, there has not been an updated projection of the urology workforce per capita beyond 2035 with updated understanding of the current urology workforce.[4] The US Department of Health and Human Services suggests that at least a decade is required to enact policy and programs to increase physician workforce, primarily because of the length of training and time required to change physician training infrastructure.[2] Therefore, it is time critical to have a nuanced understanding of the impending workforce shortage in urology per capita to mitigate the negative downstream effects in the future. Our prior study was the first to project the urologic workforce per capita and demographic of urology over the next 40 years under guided assumptions with two stock and flow models. We hypothesized that in our continued growth model, there will be a recovery beyond the current 2020 urologic workforce per capita, whereas in our stagnant growth model, we will see a continued decline in the urologic workforce per capita. We also hypothesized that the urology workforce shortage per capita will be more severe for the 65 years and older population. Lastly, we hypothesize that there will be an overall growth of female urologists per capita.

Since our original study, there has been updated information on the current urology workforce based on the AUA Census of 2021 and Accreditation Council for Graduate Medical Education (ACGME) Data Resource Book of 2021 to 2022. Additionally, given the growing concern of physician shortage, Centers for Medicare & Medicaid Services established the Consolidated Appropriations Act in 2021 that implements new Medicare-funded residency slots to qualifying hospitals of 200 slots per year over 5 years.[9] At this time, it is planned that 125 of the slots will be allocated for primary care, including obstetrics/gynecology, and 20 slots allocated to psychiatry.[9] Although the number of urology residency slots that will be supported by this new act is unclear at this time, it is promising to see specific health policy changes addressing the widespread impending physician shortage. Therefore, we have used more contemporary data for our assumptions for an updated workforce projection.

METHODS

Because we used publicly available data, our institution deemed this analysis exempt from institutional review board oversight. Informed consent was waived by our institution for this reason. This study followed the Strengthening the Reporting of Observational Studies in Epidemiology (STROBE) reporting guidelines.

Current Urologist Population

According to the 2021 AUA Census, which defines the urologist population by National Provider Identifier, valid medical licenses of urologists and pediatric urologists, and the American Board of Urology certification records, there are currently 13,790 practicing urologists consisting of 12,281 (89.1%) males and 1509 (10.9%) females.[8] It estimated that there are 4.16 urologists to 100,000 population.[8] The 2021 AUA census provided the age distribution for all practicing urologists.[8] These were used to estimate the number of practicing urologists by age and gender in 2021. Each gender and age are divided proportionally into 5-year age categories and used as the estimate of practicing urologists by gender and age group in 2021.

United States Population Data

We used the US Census Bureau 2017 national population projections based on the census data from 2010 using a cohort-component method and assumptions about demographic components of change, such as future trends in births, deaths, and net international migration from 2017 to 2060.[10]

Stock and Flow Model

The stock and flow model estimates the number of practicing urologists in a year with the addition of urology residents entering the current practicing urologist population and subtraction of the retiring urologists:

Urologist(i+1) = Urologist(i) + Residents(i)–Retirees(i), i = half-decade increment in time.

Inflow of Residents to Practice

Given that 336 urologists entered the workforce in 2022 according to the ACGME Data Resource Book, we assumed that 340 urologists would enter the workforce annually.[11] Among those entering workforce in 2022, ACGME Data Resource Book estimates that 30.4% are female, whereas the AUA Residents and Fellows Census approximates 30.9% are female.[7,11] We assume the future proportion will continue to be 30% female and 70% male and that they enter at 32 years.[8] For the continued growth model, we assumed growth rate of 37.6% every 5 years of increasing number of urologists entering the workforce using the ACGME growth rate from 2017 to 2022.[11] For the stagnant growth model, the number of incoming urologists remained at 340.

Outflow of Urologists Through Retirement

The flow portion of the model subtracts the retiring urologists from the population using the 2021 AUA Census. The 2021 AUA Census provided the proportion of urologists in 5-year increments of planned age at full retirement separated by gender. Based on the stable planned retirement age in AUA census from 2016 to 2021, we assumed that these retirement proportions would remain constant throughout the time projected.[8,12–15]

Per Capita

The per capita estimates are calculated using the estimated urologist population and dividing by the US population. We calculated total urologists, male urologists, and female urologist per total capita. We also calculated per greater than or equal to 65 years population and urologists per matching gender per capita. Stock and flow models were generated in Microsoft-Excel (2016).

RESULTS

In 2021, according to the AUA census, there were 13,790 total practicing urologists with 12,281 (89.1%) being male and 1509 (10.9%) being female. Our assumptions for the study are listed in **Table 1**. The median age of urologists was 54 years.

Accounting for the incoming urologist workforce graduating from residency and the outflow of retiring urologists, our continued growth model predicted that 2027 will have the lowest number of urologists at 12,296; the workforce will recover to baseline 2022 levels by 2037 with 15,015 urologists (**Fig. 1**). The total number of female urologists will grow 7.67-fold from 2022 to 2057 with an absolute increase of 10,756 urologists. In 2057, we anticipate 12,369 female urologists, which will comprise 29.8% of total urology workforce. Comparatively, the total number of male urologists will grow 2.39-fold from 2022 to 2057 with an absolute increase of 16,594 urologists. The total absolute growth of female urologists is 39.3% of the total absolute growth of male urologists from 2022 to 2057. The median age of urology workforce peaks at 50 to 54 years in 2022, and then will downtrend to 40 to 44 years by 2037. We anticipate the median age range of female urology workforce members to be 40 to 44 years through 2057. Comparatively, the median age range of male urology workforce members is at its peak of 55 to 59 years in 2022 and will downtrend to 40 to 44 years by 2042.

In our stagnant growth model, the year 2027 will have the lowest number of urologists at 12,168;

Table 1
Key forecast assumptions

Variable	Key Assumption	Sources
Baseline practicing urologists	13,790	2021 AUA Census
Male vs female practicing urologists, n (%)	Male, 12,281 (89.1) Female, 1509 (10.9)	2021 AUA Census
Practicing urologists, age (median)	54 y	2021 AUA Census
Age of male vs female new urologists annually	32 y	2021 AUA Census
Baseline new annual urologists	340 (vs 336 on ACGME 2022)	ACGME workbook 2022
Graduating resident, growth per 5 y	0% baseline growth 37.6% baseline growth	ACGME workbook 2022 From 2017 to 2022, 37.6% growth
New urologists annually that are female, %	30 (vs 30.4 on ACGME 2022; 30.9 AUA 2021)	2021 AUA Census, 2022 ACGME
Age of male vs female planned age of retirement (median)	Male, 68 y Female, 65 y	2021 AUA Census

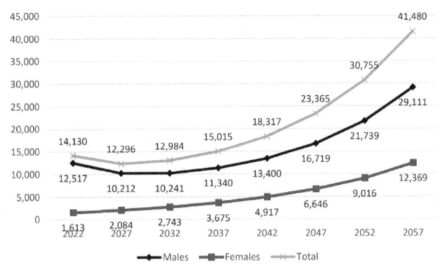

Fig. 1. Projected number of urologists and their demographics with continued (37.6%) growth in the urology resident workforce every 5 years (total vs male vs female).

the workforce will not recover to baseline 2022 levels, instead only reaching 12,866 by 2057 (**Fig. 2**). The total number of female urologists will grow 2.26-fold from 2022 to 2057 with an absolute increase of 2036 urologists. The total number of male urologists will decrease by 26.4% from 2022 to 2057 with an absolute decrease of 3301 urologists. The median age of urology workforce peaks to 50 to 54 years in 2022, and then will downtrend to 45 to 49 years by 2027. We anticipate the median age range of female urology workforce members to be 40 to 44 years through 2037, and 45 to 49 years from 2042 on. Comparatively, the median age range of male urology workforce members is at its peak of 55 to 59 years in 2022 and will downtrend to 50 to 54 years by 2027.

In our continued growth model of 37.6% more urologists joining practice every 5 years, 2027 will have the lowest urologists per capita of 3.5 urologists per 100,000 persons (**Fig. 3**). By 2057, there will be 10.4 urologists per 100,000 persons. For the Medicare population, there are currently 23.7 urologists per 100,000 persons greater than or equal to 65 years in 2020 (**Fig. 4**). This ratio is the lowest in 2032 with 17.3 urologists per 100,000 persons greater than or equal to 65 years, which increases to 45.2 by 2057. When matching female urologists to the female population, there are 0.9 female urologists to 100,000 female persons in 2022, which increases at each time interval to 6.1 female urologists to 100,000 female persons by 2057 (**Fig. 5**).

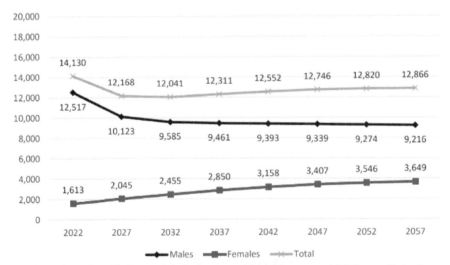

Fig. 2. Projected number of urologists and their demographics with stagnant (0%) growth in the urology resident workforce every 5 years (total vs male vs female).

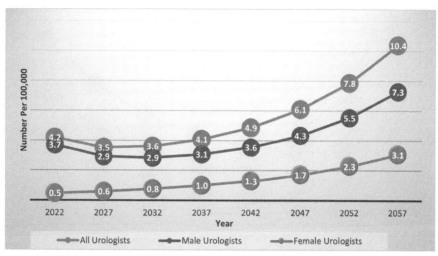

Fig. 3. Projected number of urologists per capita from 2022 to 2057 with continued (37.6%) growth in the urology resident workforce every 5 years (all urologists, male urologists, female urologists).

In our stagnant growth model of 0%, there will be a continued decrease of urologists per capita to 3.2 urologists per 100,000 persons in 2057 (**Fig. 6**). For the Medicare population, there is a continued decrease at each time point with 14.0 urologists per 100,000 persons greater than or equal to 65 years by 2057 (**Fig. 7**). When matching female urologists to the female population, there is continued growth that plateaus at 4.1 female urologists to 100,000 female persons in 2047 and beyond (**Fig. 8**).

DISCUSSION

Our updated projection of the urologic workforce per capita and demographics of urology over the next 40 years has four key findings. First, median age range of female urology workforce is significantly younger than the male cohort, which contributes to the decline in the median age range of overall urology workforce in the coming decades. Second, the total number of practicing urologists per capita will decrease over the next decade, even with sustained growth of the resident complement across urology training programs and will not recover to baseline until 2042. Third, there will be a prolonged shortage of total urologists per greater than or equal to 65 years populations in both models compared with the overall population in both our projection models. Finally, female urologists per capita will continue to increase in the context of decreasing urologists per capita in

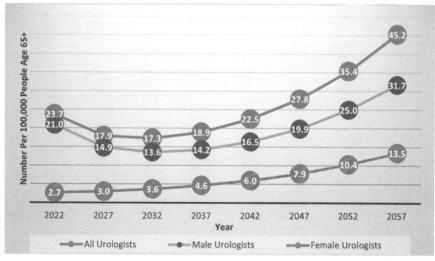

Fig. 4. Projected number of urologists per 100,000 people aged 65 years or older with continued (37.6%) growth in the urology resident workforce every 5 years from 2022 to 2057 (all urologists, male urologists, female urologists).

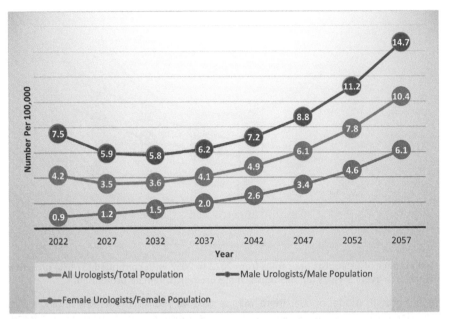

Fig. 5. Projected number of urologists per capita by matching gender with continued (37.6%) growth in the urology resident workforce every 5 years from 2022 to 2057 (all urologists per capita, male urologists per male population, female urologists per female population).

continued growth and stagnant growth models. Collectively, these projections highlight the severity of the impending shortage of urologists and importance of structural change and advocacy to maximize our available urologic workforce, particularly the female urologists that constitute a large portion of this urologic workforce.

Although the median age of the urology workforce was 52.5 years in 2009, it is 54 years in 2021.[15,16] In contrast, the female median age

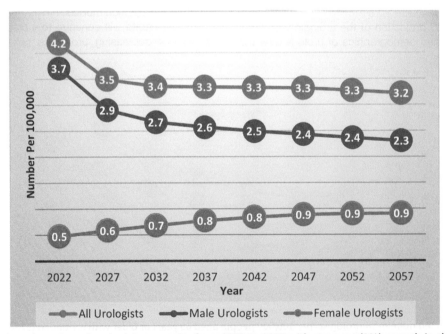

Fig. 6. Projected number of urologists per capita from 2022 to 2057 with stagnant (0%) growth in the urology resident workforce every 5 years (all urologists, male urologists, female urologists).

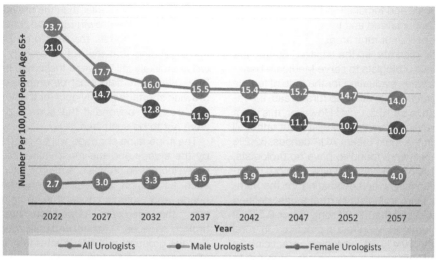

Fig. 7. Projected number of urologists per 100,000 people aged 65 years or older with stagnant (0%) growth in the urology resident workforce every 5 years from 2022 to 2057 (all urologists, male urologists, female urologists).

range is significantly younger at 40 to 44 years in 2022 and continues to hover in that range throughout our projections for both models. With the impending retirement for about a quarter of practicing urologists, it is important to understand what practices will be most impacted by retirement in the coming decades. Gaither and colleagues[17] studied the retirement pattern of the urologic workforce using the AUA 2014 census and found that urologists near retirement tend to practice general urology in a solo practice outside of metropolitan areas. As these practicing urologists near retirement and scale down their clinical practice, there will be exaggerated gaps of care in nonmetropolitan and solo practice areas. Given that there is significant growth of female urologists concurrently, it is likely that some of this supply gap will be filled by female urologists. Our current understanding of female urologists' practice patterns, however, is that when compared with men, they are subspecialized, at academic centers, and in metropolitan areas.[18,19] Similarly, young

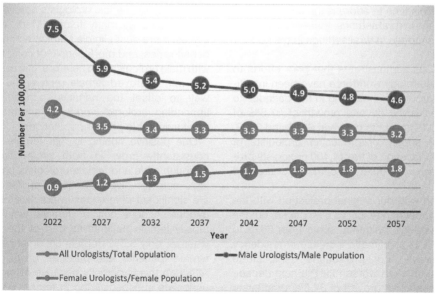

Fig. 8. Projected number of urologists per capita by matching gender with stagnant (0%) growth in urology resident workforce every 5 years from 2022 to 2057 (all urologists, male urologists per male population, female urologists per female population).

urologists, male and female, tend to be dispropor-tionately subspecialized and less likely to practice in nonmetropolitan or rural areas.[18,20] One-third of the hospital markets in the United States are without female urologists to serve Medicare bene-ficiaries and when evaluating for the ratio of female urologists practicing in urban to rural areas, the ra-tio was found to be 16.5:1.[18,21] However, this is not an issue specific to female urologists, but rather all urologists. In the most recent AUA census, 62.2% of US counties were found to have no urologists, and only 11% of counties had nine or more urolo-gists.[8] Additionally, when evaluating for the num-ber of practicing urologists in rural areas, defined as population less than 2500, only 63 or 0.5% of the overall urologic workforce practices in rural settings with 10.4% of urologists practicing in nonmetropolitan areas, defined as population less than 50,000.[8] More concerning is that older urologists were more often found to be practicing in nonmetropolitan areas compared with younger urologists.[8] Therefore, the gap of urologic work-force left behind by retiring urologists is less likely to be filled by female or young urologists in the future without changes in their practice patterns or policy changes encouraging urologists to prac-tice in rural settings. One example is the Specialty Physicians Advancing Rural Care Act (SPARC Act), which has been introduced by Senator Rosen and proposes student loan repayment programs to support specialty medical care in rural areas. This can potentially draw younger urologists to fill urologist gaps to practice in rural or nonmetropol-itan areas. If we do not make meaningful policy changes at this time to address the urology work-force shortage in rural settings, there will likely be a worsening shortage in rural settings in the coming decades.

Our analysis demonstrates that prior efforts to increase the urology workforce have been insuffi-cient, with problems escalating in the decades to come. Specifically, despite growth of 37.6% of urology residency spots between 2017 and 2022, the current supply of practicing urologists of 13,790 is still far short of the 14,400 urologists pro-jected necessary to meet the demand for urologic services.[2,11]

Compared with our original projection with the continued growth rate of 13.8% based on the growth of urology residency spots from 2013 to 2018, 37.6% is a dramatic increase in residency spots. However, our projections demonstrate that the disparity will worsen for the next decade even with continued growth of 37.6% graduating urologists every 5 years.[2] Because of the number of retiring urologists, the number of providers per capita will not reach baseline 2022 levels until 2042, which is still earlier than the previous projec-tion with the lower growth rate. We provided these two alternate models for workforce projections, understanding that the actual urology workforce will most likely fall between these two projections. Regardless, the field must be prepared to face a growing shortage of providers for the next decade, and possibly beyond if the current growth rate were not to be sustained.

The impending shortage will be felt most keenly by the elderly and the most vulnerable patients. Given increased prevalence of urologic conditions, such as benign prostatic hyperplasia, inconti-nence, and urologic cancers, in an aging popula-tion, the Medicare population heavily uses urology services.[16] Etzioni and colleagues[22] found that the group of patients greater than or equal to 65 years used 64.8% of all urologic services. McKibben and colleagues[4] reaffirmed that adults greater than or equal to 65 years use urologic ser-vices at a rate three-times higher than the general population. Both of our models show a decline in urologists per 100,000 persons greater than or equal to 65 years in the coming years, which is particularly concerning given that this population heavily uses urology services, thereby exacer-bating the existing shortage of urologist supply relative to the demand.[4] This has significant down-stream consequences on access to care, delays for surgical evaluation, and potential for worse pa-tient outcomes.[23] Increasing diversity among health care providers, however, has been associ-ated with improved access for underserved popu-lations and more research into health disparities.[24] Within urology, female urologists have been found to see twice as many female Medicare benefi-ciaries, more dual-eligible Medicare and Medicaid beneficiaries, and more people of color compared with male urologists.[21] Therefore, increasing diver-sity with improved female representation is one way to offset the negative consequences of impending urologic workforce shortage on the most vulnerable patient populations.

One positive finding is that female urologists consistently grow in both projection models. Although male and female urologists provide uro-logic care for diverse patient populations, there are significant differences in practice patterns by gender. Almost half of female urologists see mostly female patients as part of their practice, whereas only 3.5% of male urologists see mostly female patients as part of their practice.[13] Although this is partially because of more female urologists subspecializing in female pelvic medi-cine and reconstructive surgery, when comparing general urologists of each gender, female general urologists logged 2.2 times the number of urogynecologic cases compared with their male counterparts.[25,26] Currently, with 0.9 female urologists per 100,000 female population, there is significant underrepresentation of female urologists for a gender-concordant population in the United States. In our continued growth model, 6.1 female urologists per 100,000 female population has been projected by 2057, which is still lower than the current male urologists per 100,000 male population in 2022, which further contextualizes how underrepresented female urologists are for gender-concordant population in the United States. This is particularly noteworthy given that 30% of urologic patients are female and patient surveys have highlighted patient preference for gender-concordant urologists for urinary incontinence.[27] With an increasing number of female urologists in our projection, they have not only increased availability to provide care for female patients but also increase the likelihood of mutually respective care for diverse patient populations by contributing to the diversity of the urologic workforce.[5] Additionally, female physicians add value to health care organizations and to patients by being more likely to practice evidence-based medicine, associated with lower risk of death, readmission, or postoperative complication with comparable or improved postoperative outcomes when compared with male physicians.[24,28–32] Therefore, regardless of the gender of the patient, patients will likely benefit from increasing representation of female urologists.

As female urologists contribute more heavily to the overall urologic workforce, there have been concerns regarding whether female urologists work less than male urologists since female physicians across specialties have been found to work 7.4 hours less than male physicians per week.[33] Several studies within urology, however, found that after adjusting for age, practice type, subspecialty, and inpatient operations performed, there were no difference in hours worked between male and female urologists.[34–36] Therefore, current data do not support the hypothesis of worsening urologic workforce shortage because of female urologists working fewer hours compared with male counterparts.

Our study has several limitations. The projections of the workforce model are dependent on assumptions listed in **Table 1**. Although the current urology resident workforce consists of 30% female, which is significantly higher than previously, we did not think that this growth in representation would be linear. Therefore, we assumed that about 30% of the resident workforce will be female, understanding that this could likely be an underestimate. For the newly graduated urology residents

joining the workforce, we assumed that board certification rate between male and female would be comparable and that the average age of entering the workforce is 32 years for both male and female. We also used planned retirement age as a surrogate for actual retirement age because that was the closest data we had available. There are limited longitudinal data that exist for some of our assumptions, but the two scenarios of continued and stagnant growth were modeled to account for possible variability, understanding that the actual urology workforce will most likely fall between these two models. Our second limitation is that our projections consist of the total number of urologists in practice and their demographics, but they are not representative of their full-time equivalents. We believed that we would focus on the total number of practicing urologists to provide a broad understanding of the upcoming urology workforce in the coming decades given that there are also limitations with extrapolating the current full-time equivalents data in our projection. Third, we cannot account for the changes to urologist's changes in retirement plans with the increasing number of urologists. Given that approximately 10% of the urologists continue to practice because of their inability to recruit a replacement, if there are more urologists available, they may plan to retire earlier.[15]

These limitations notwithstanding, our findings stress the time sensitivity and importance of training additional urologists and supporting currently practicing urologists to ensure that we effectively mitigate the impending urology workforce shortage. For practicing urologists, our findings are relevant in how they adjust their practice patterns. Urologists may increase their practice hours or hire more advanced practice providers (APPs). Although APPs have been vital partners in providing quality care to patients and potentially bridge the gap between patient's access to care, it is crucial for the number of urologists to grow alongside the APPs given that urologists are crucial in delivering surgical services and the extent of APP's practice within urology is currently understudied.[4] Another possible adaptation is increasing the foothold of telemedicine to make urologists be able to reach more rural areas and increase clinical efficiency. However, it is still largely unknown whether video visits can substitute clinic evaluations and how it affects clinical efficacy.[37,38]

Our findings also highlight the necessity of institutional and national policy changes to ensure a supportive work environment for female urologists, who will heavily consist of the absolute growth of urologists for the next four decades. First, stronger recruitment efforts are needed to ensure that there is a strong urology pipeline into the future. Although we have seen tremendous growth of female urologists in our field, Findlay and colleagues[39] found that when looking at the annual rate of change in increase in female representation, urology ranked eighth out of nine surgical specialties, which is concerning for slowing growth in the trainee pipeline. Recruitment efforts are especially critical for female medical students, given that urology continues to be male dominated and female medical students who pursue urology are also more likely to report discrimination, abuse, or harassment compared with male applicants.[40] We must do better to identify and eliminate these behaviors to make urology more inclusive toward female trainees. The strong recruitment will likely have positive downstream consequences with further recruitment of female medical students into the field given that positive correlation between the proportion of matched female applicants and female proportion of residents.[41]

Second, urology as a field needs to make it more feasible to achieve pregnancy and parenthood as a urologist if he or she were to desire it. Multiple studies have demonstrated that female surgeons use assisted reproductive technologies and experience major pregnancy-related complications at higher rates compared with the general population.[42–45] Therefore, there needs to be institutional and national policy changes to help support pregnancy and parenthood. The American Board of Medical Specialties recommended a minimum of 6 weeks of parental, caregiver, or medical leave without exhausting other allowed time away.[46] Therefore, the American Board of Urology proposed a more flexible model of "averaging" the 46-week requirement over the last 2 years of training, which allows trainees to get protected leave while also progressing toward independent practice during the final 2 years of residency.[46] A natural extension of this policy change would be to include infrastructural changes to help support parental leave for practicing urologists.[47] In one survey, practicing surgeons, male and female, reported that they desired longer parental leave and most did not have designated parental or family leave policy in their contract, and had to rely on short-term disability or personal savings during their leave.[48] Although parenthood is traditionally thought to be a female issue, having young children has been associated with lower work-life balance satisfaction among urologists, male and female.[49] Therefore, it is important to reframe and address the challenges of parenthood as early career urologists and beyond to prevent burnout and maximize well-being among urologists.

Third, we must address the gender pay gap in urology. Gender pay gap persists across all medical subspecialties and a recent study evaluating the career differences of income between men and women physicians found gross income difference of $2 million over a 40-year career, with largest differences found in surgical specialists of $2.5 million.[50] In urology, female gender was a predictor for lower compensation with adjusted salaries being $76,321 less than male urologists while controlling for work hours, call frequency, age, practice setting and type, fellowship training, and advance practice provider employment.[35] Vollstedt and coworkers[51] reviewed strategies that had been proposed to address the gender pay gap including reevaluating wRVU system given that female surgeons are more likely to perform surgeries associated with lower wRVU value and wRVU does not correlate well with surgical complexity or work effort. Some other examples include faculty salary equity review committee to narrow the gender pay gap, pay transparency, and salary-only compensation models.[51]

Fourth, we need to address the leaky pipeline. Although physician burnout remains a constant threat to a stable urologist workforce, it could affect male and female urologists differently. For example, AUA Workforce workgroup recently compared the rate of burnout of urologists from AUA Census of 2016 to 2021.[52] They found that whereas the rate of burnout decreased in men from 36.3% to 35.2% over these 5 years, women's burnout increased from 35.3% to 49.2% over the same time period.[52] Although burnout is likely multifactorial and complex, one possible contributor is that female physicians have been found to spend an average of 8.5 additional hours per week on domestic activities compared with their male counterparts.[53] This is particularly striking in the context of female physicians being more likely to be married to full-time working professionals and yet female physicians are still more likely to be primarily responsible for domestic chores.[53–56] Creating organizational culture where urologists are supported through greater autonomy and flexibility, improvements in work-life balance, more diverse and inclusive work communities, and greater efficiency will help buffer against burnout and lead to a more robust, stable, and productive workforce. One example is sick-child day care instituted by the Mayo Clinic after recognizing that the hospital, on average, lost half day of work per employee annually because of lack of a back-up childcare system.[57] Mayo Clinic found that the saved workdays offset the operational costs of setting up a sick-child day care center.[57] Another example is a time-banking program established by Stanford University School of Medicine, where it recognizes work activities that are typically not recognized, such as mentoring, sitting on a committee, or filling in last minute for a colleague.[58] These activities are then converted to credits, which can be used in the future for work or home activities, which allows additional flexibility for physicians.[58]

Additionally, the increasing representation of female urologists should also be reflected by a growing number of women in leadership roles, which will lead to increased visibility of women at academic centers and improved access to mentorship for female medical students and residents.[18] Mentorship continues to be important in a female urologist's career, where a recent survey found that younger female faculty found having a gender-concordant mentor in the same department or institution to be critical.[18] This is a challenge when there are promotion disparities in academic urology. Breyer and colleagues[24,59] found that on average, women took 1.2 years longer than men to advance from assistant to associate professor even when controlling for age, years since residency, publications, and grants. Female urologists also have higher attrition in academic practice compared with male urologists.[24] Although this is likely multifactorial, there could be institutional or national policies to ameliorate such promotion disparity and promote faculty retention. One example is "clock stopping," where an institution does not include period of maternity leave and portion of pregnancy in terms of meeting publication quota as part of promotion evaluation.[54,55,60] Another example is the Diversity and Inclusion task force of AUA or professional societies, such as the Society of Women in Urology, which has made a concerted effort to recognize women for AUA awards and to nominate and promote women for leadership positions.[32]

SUMMARY

In our projection of the urology workforce to 2057, female urologists make up a significant proportion of the workforce growth over the next four decades in both models. The median age range of the female urology workforce is significantly younger than the male cohort, which contributes to an overall decline median age range of the urology workforce in the coming decades. Given the length of training and time required to change physician training infrastructure, there is an urgent need for advocacy to increase graduate medical education funding to train more urologists to mitigate this shortage, and structural changes to support female urologists.

CLINICS CARE POINTS

- In our projection of the urology workforce to 2057, female urologists make up a significant portion of the workforce growth over the next four decades in both continued and stagnant growth models.
- Given the length of training and time required to change physician training infrastructure, there is an urgent need for advocacy to mitigate this shortage.
- Some examples include more recruitment efforts for a strong urology pipeline, policy changes to make it more feasible to achieve pregnancy and parenthood as a urologist, address the gender pay gap in urology, and address the leaky pipeline.

DISCLOSURE

No commercial or financial conflicts of interest or funding sources for all authors.

REFERENCES

1. Williams TE, Satiani B, Thomas A, et al. The impending shortage and the estimated cost of training the future surgical workforce. Ann Surg 2009;250(4):590–6. https://doi.org/10.1097/SLA.0b013e3181b6c90b.
2. Physician Supply and Demand, *Projections to 2020*. *U.S. Departmentof Health and Human Services Health Resources;* 2006. Available at: http://bhw.hrsa.gov/sites/default/files/bhw/nchwa/projections/physician 2020-projections.pdf. Accessed January 30, 2023.
3. American Urological Association. Our priority: address the urologic workforce shortage. Available at: https://www.auanet.org/advocacy/federal-advocacy/workforce-shortages. Accessed January 30, 2023.
4. McKibben MJ, Kirby EW, Langston J, et al. Projecting the urology workforce over the next 20 years. Urology 2016;98:21–6.
5. Halpern JA, Lee UJ, Wolff EM, et al. Women in urology residency, 1978-2013: a critical look at gender representation in our specialty. Urology 2016;92:20–5.
6. Holton MR, Bailey K. Women in urology. Urol Clin 2021;48(2):187–94.
7. Urologists in Training: Residents &Fellows in the United States. American Urological Association 2020-2021. Available at: https://www.auanet.org/documents/research/census/DAT-22-7794%20Residents_Fellows %20Census%20Report.pdf. Accessed January 30, 2023.
8. The State of the Urology Workforce and Practice in the United States. 2021. Available at: https://www.AUAnet.org/common/pdf/. Accessed January 30, 2023.

9. CMS Awards 200 New Medicare-Funded Residency Slots to Hospitals Serving Underserved Communities; 2023. Available at: https://www.cms.gov/newsroom/press-releases/cms-awards-200-new-medicare-funded-residency-slots-hospitals-serving-under served-communities. Accessed January 30, 2023.

10. Methodology, Assumptions, and Inputs for the 2017 National Population Projections.; 2018. Available at: https://www2.census.gov/programs-surveys/pop proj/technical-documentation/methodology/method statement17.pdf. Accessed January 30, 2023.

11. Accreditation Council For Graduate Medical Education Book Resource Data. Available at: www.acgme.org. Accessed January 30, 2023.

12. The State of the Urology Workforce and Practice in the United States. 2020. Available at: https://www.auanet.org/documents/research/census/2020-State-of-Urology-Workforce-Census-Book.pdf. Accessed January 30, 2023.

13. The State of the Urology Workforce and Practice in the United States.; 2018. Available at: https://www.AUAnet.org/common/pdf/. Accessed January 30, 2023.

14. The State of the Urology Workforce and Practice in the United States.; 2016. Available at: www.AUAnet.org/TakeCensus. Accessed January 30, 2023.

15. The State of the Urology Workforce and Practice in the United States. 2019. Available at: https://www.auanet.org/documents/research/census/2019%20The%20State%20of%20the%20Urology%20Work force%20Census%20Book.pdf. Accessed January 30, 2023.

16. Pruthi RS, Neuwahl S, Nielsen ME, et al. Recent trends in the urology workforce in the United States. Urology 2013;82(5):987–94.

17. Gaither TW, Awad MA, Fang R, et al. The near-future impact of retirement on the urologic workforce: results from the American Urological Association census. Urology 2016;94:85–9.

18. Saltzman A, Hebert K, Richman A, et al. Women urologists: changing trends in the workforce. Urology 2016;91:1–5.

19. Tsugawa Y, Jena AB, Figueroa JF, et al. Comparison of hospital mortality and readmission rates for Medicare patients treated by male vs female physicians. JAMA Intern Med 2017;177(2):206–13.

20. Nettey OS, Fuchs JS, Kielb SJ, et al. Gender representation in urologic subspecialties. Urology 2018; 114:66–70.

21. Nam CS, Mehta A, Hammett J, et al. Variation in practice patterns and reimbursements between female and male urologists for Medicare beneficiaries. JAMA Netw Open 2019. https://doi.org/10.1001/jamanetworkopen.2019.8956.

22. Etzioni DA, Liu JH, Maggard MA, et al. The aging population and its impact on the surgery workforce. Ann Surg 2003;238(2):170–7.

23. Mahoney ST, Strassle PD, Schroen AT, et al. Survey of the US surgeon workforce: practice characteristics, job satisfaction, and reasons for leaving surgery. J Am Coll Surg 2020;230:283–93.e1. Elsevier Inc.

24. Malik RD, Salles A. Debunking four common gender equity myths. Eur Urol 2022;81(6):552–4.

25. Liu JS, Dickmeyer LJ, Nettey O, et al. Disparities in female urologic case distribution with new subspecialty certification and surgeon gender. Neurourol Urodyn 2017;36(2):399–403.

26. Rotker K, Iosifescu S, Baird G, et al. What's gender got to do with it: difference in the proportion of traditionally female cases performed by general urologists of each gender. Urology 2018;116:35–40.

27. Ficko Z, Li Z, Hyams ES. Urology is a sensitive area: assessing patient preferences for male or female urologists. Urol Pract 2018;5(2):139–42.

28. Wallis CJ, Ravi B, Coburn N, et al. Comparison of postoperative outcomes among patients treated by male and female surgeons: a population based matched cohort study. BMJ (Online) 2017;359. https://doi.org/10.1136/bmj.j4366.

29. Sharoky CE, Sellers MM, Keele LJ, et al. Does surgeon sex matter practice patterns and outcomes of female and male surgeons. Ann Surg 2018; 267(6):1069–76.

30. Parks AL, Redberg RF. Women in medicine and patient outcomes equal rights for better work? JAMA Intern Med 2017;177(2):161.

31. Wallis CJD, Jerath A, Coburn N, et al. Association of surgeon-patient sex concordance with postoperative outcomes. JAMA Surg 2022;157(2):146–56.

32. Mehta A. Challenges facing women in sexual medicine. J Sex Med 2022;19(10):1502–5.

33. HEALTH CARE REFORM Annual Work Hours Across Physician Specialties. Available at: http://www.archinternmed.com. Accessed January 30, 2023.

34. Porten SP, Gaither TW, Greene KL, et al. Do women work less than men in urology: data from the American Urological Association census. Urology 2018; 118:71–5.

35. Spencer ES, Deal AM, Pruthi NR, et al. Gender differences in compensation, job satisfaction and other practice patterns in urology. J Urol 2016;195(2):450–5.

36. Lightner DJ, Terris MK, Tsao AK, et al. Status of women in urology: based on a report to the society of university urologists. J Urol 2005;173(2):560–3.

37. Andino JJ, Castaneda PR, Shah PK, et al. The impact of video visits on measures of clinical efficiency and reimbursement. Urol Pract 2021;8(1):53–7.

38. Andino JJ, Lingaya MA, Daignault-Newton S, et al. Video visits as a substitute for urological clinic visits. Urology 2020;144:46–51.

39. Findlay BL, Bearrick EN, Granberg CF, et al. Path to parity: trends in female representation among physicians, trainees, and applicants in urology and

surgical specialties. Urology 2022. https://doi.org/10.1016/j.urology.2022.11.033.

40. Wong D, Kuprasertkul A, Khouri RK, et al. Assessing the female and underrepresented minority medical student experience in the urology match: where do we fall short? Urology 2021;147:57–63.

41. Kapur A, Hung M, Wang K, et al. The future is female: the influence of female faculty and resident representation on female applicant match rate amongst urology residency programs over 3 years. Urology 2022;160:46–50.

42. Rangel EL, Castillo-Angeles M, Easter SR, et al. Incidence of infertility and pregnancy complications in US female surgeons. JAMA Surg 2021;156(10):905–15.

43. Atkinson RB, Castillo-Angeles M, Kim ES, et al. The long road to parenthood assisted reproduction, surrogacy, and adoption among US surgeons. Ann Surg 2022;275(1):106–14.

44. Rangel EL, Smink DS, Castillo-Angeles M, et al. Pregnancy and motherhood during surgical training. JAMA Surg 2018;153(7):644–52.

45. Rangel EL, Lyu H, Haider AH, et al. Factors associated with residency and career dissatisfaction in childbearing surgical residents. JAMA Surg 2018;153(11):1004–11.

46. Greenberg R, Thavaseelan S, Mary, Westerman B. ABMS Releases New Parental and Caregiver Leave Policy, ABU Responds. Available at: https://www.auanet.org/membership/publications-overview/aua-news/all-articles/2021/april-2021/abms-releases-new-parental-and-caregiver-leave-policy-abu-responds. Accessed January 30, 2023.

47. Stephens EH, Heisler CA, Temkin SM, et al. The current status of women in surgery: how to affect the future. JAMA Surg 2020;155(9):876–85.

48. Gaines T, Harkhani N, Chen H, et al. Current policies and practicing surgeon perspectives on parental leave. Am J Surg 2019;218(4):772–9.

49. Nam CS, Daignault-Newton S, Herrel LA, et al. Can you have it all? Parenting in urology and work-life balance satisfaction. Urology 2023. https://doi.org/10.1016/j.urology.2022.12.044.

50. Whaley CM, Koo T, Arora VM, et al. Female physicians earn an estimated $2 million less than male physicians over a simulated 40-year career. Health Aff 2021;40(12):1856–64.

51. Vollstedt A, Hougen HY, Gupta P, et al. Gender-based pay gap in urology: a review of the literature and potential solutions. Urology 2022;168:21–6.

52. Harris AM, Teplitsky S, Kraft KH, et al. Burnout: a call to action from the AUA workforce workgroup. J Urol 2023. https://doi.org/10.1097/JU.0000000000003108.

53. Jolly S, Griffith KA, DeCastro R, et al. Gender differences in time spent on parenting and domestic responsibilities by high-achieving young physician-researchers. Ann Intern Med 2014;160(5):344–53.

54. Baptiste D, Fecher AM, Dolejs SC, et al. Gender differences in academic surgery, work-life balance, and satisfaction. J Surg Res 2017;218:99–107.

55. Johnson HM, Irish W, Strassle PD, et al. Associations between career satisfaction, personal life factors, and work-life integration practices among US surgeons by gender. JAMA Surg 2020;155(8):742–50.

56. Streu R, McGrath MH, Gay A, et al. Plastic surgeons' satisfaction with work-life balance: results from a national survey. Plast Reconstr Surg 2011;127(4):1713–9.

57. Snyder RA, Tarpley MJ, Phillips SE, et al. The case for on-site child care in residency training and afterward. J Grad Med Educ 2013;5(3):365–7.

58. Berg S, Bookmark MR. Working Overtime? At Stanford, Physicians Bank the Time for Later.; 2018. Available at: https://www.ama-assn.org/practice-management/physician-health/working-overtime-stanford-physicians-bank-time-later. Accessed January 30, 2023.

59. Breyer BN, Butler C, Fang R, et al. Promotion disparities in academic urology. Urology 2020;138:16–23.

60. MacDonald SM, Malik RD. Women in academic urology: a qualitative analysis of the relationship between pregnancy, parenting, and delayed promotion. Urology 2022;168:13–20.

Experiences of Diverse Providers

The Gender Gap in Promotions
Inhibitors and Catalysts, Strategies to Close the Gap

Susan M. MacDonald, MD[a,*], Rena D. Malik, MD[b]

KEYWORDS

• Gender disparity • Gender bias • Academic urology • Academic surgery • Promotion

KEY POINTS

- In the workplace, women's chances of career advancement are diminished by objective indicators, such as lower compensation, lower research funding, fewer leadership and speaking opportunities, and a disproportionate allocation of time toward clinical duties and administrative tasks.
- Lack of transparent promotional criteria, increased time spent in citizenship duties, time for maternity leave and lactation, combating gender bias, decreased networking opportunities, and decreased availability of same-sex mentorship/sponsorship further compound these obstacles.
- Strategies to narrow the gender gap in promotions include: 1) creating programs with funding and staff dedicated to supporting women and marginalized groups, 2) establishing transparent criteria for promotion, leadership selection, and compensation 3) developing standard, equitable expectations for citizenship duties and low-acuity tasks for all faculty and 4) implementing ongoing DEI education programs with trackable outcomes.

BACKGROUND

Traditionally urology has been a male-dominated specialty; just 2 years ago in the 2020 census did women surpass 10% of the workforce.[1] It seems that despite a larger number of women trainees graduating every year, there is still a lag in women reaching the upper echelons of the academic ladder and leadership within urology. In a study comparing male and female graduates from the 50 top urology programs according to US News and World report between 2002 and 2008 women were more likely to be assistant professors as compared with their male colleagues (69.4% vs 39.4%) and fewer had been promoted to associate (27.8% vs 48.9%) or full professor (2.8% vs 11.7%).[2] Breyer and colleagues[3] examined the American Urological Association (AUA) 2017 census data and found that women were delayed promotion to associate professor (7.3 years; 95% confidence interval [CI], 6.8–7.8), as compared with their male colleagues (6.1 years; 95% CI, 5.8–6.6). Furthermore, men were twice as likely to be promoted to associate professor within 4 years compared with women in their multivariable analysis (odds ratio, 2.3; $P = .008$).[3] This disparity in urology is emblematic of a systemic problem in academic medicine as Richter and Clark[4] demonstrated with data from the Association of American Medical Colleges of medical school graduates from 1979 to 2013. Across all specialties in medicine women were 24% less like likely to be promoted to associate professor than men, 23% less likely to be promoted to full professor, and 54% less likely to be appointed department chair.[4]

[a] Department of Urology, Penn State Health Milton S. Hershey Medical Center, Mail Code H055, 500 University Drive, Hershey, PA 17033, USA; [b] Division of Urology, VA Long Beach Health System, 5901 East 7th Street, Long Beach, CA 90822, USA
* Corresponding author.
E-mail address: smacdonald@pennstatehealth.psu.edu

Urol Clin N Am 50 (2023) 515–524
https://doi.org/10.1016/j.ucl.2023.07.001

Women are cognizant of this disadvantage; in the 2018 AUA census 30.1% of women compared with 0.2% of men answered that their professional growth is limited by their gender.[5] This delay in promotion for women is particularly salient because nearly half the women in practice (45%) work at academic medical centers.[1] We must identify the contributing causes of delayed promotion for women in urology and actively work to combat these factors.

Identifying the cause for delayed promotion is challenging because it is multifactorial. Contributing factors include

- Poor transparency: Criteria are not clearly outlined
- Institutional variability: Criteria vary significantly between institutions
- Individual variability: Criteria are not uniformly applied between individuals at the same institution
- Lack of autonomy: Persons applying for promotion have little autonomy or personal advocacy in their own promotional process

In this article we subdivide gender disparity that impedes promotion into experiences in the workplace and outside the workplace. Furthermore, disparities within the workplace are divided into those than can be directly quantified versus those more qualitative, nebulous differences.

WORKPLACE: QUANTIFIABLE GENDER DISPARITY
Salary Inequality

Salary inequalities in academic medicine can create significant barriers to career advancement, by signaling lower levels of experience, limiting access to resources and opportunities, and reducing motivation and engagement among faculty. Gender disparities in compensation within urology have been consistently and objectively identified across multiple studies. In 1993 Bradbury and colleagues[6] surveyed women urologists and found the mean reported salary to be 65% of the national average for practicing urologists; this study, however, did not account for hours worked or academic versus private practice. In 2005 Lightner and colleagues[7] commented on the Medical Group Management Association annual financial survey, which excluded academic medical centers, and reported a mean compensation of $196,000 for women, a mere 66% of the $294,000 for men. More recently, Spencer and colleagues[8] identified a $76,321 salary discrepancy based on gender despite adjusting for hours worked, amount of call, age, practice type, and

setting. North and colleagues[9] examined the 2017 AUA census data and found that men were twice as likely to make more than $350,000 a year despite similar hours worked (**Fig. 1**).

In addition to reduced baseline income, women also receive less ancillary income from industry relationships that offer opportunities, such as networking, collaborative publications, and increased visibility, all of which enhance one's promotion portfolio. Spencer and colleagues[8] reported that female urologists were less likely to report ancillary income than men (30.1% vs 42.9%; $P = .04$). In regards to industry, a study by Velez and colleagues[10] using the Open Payments Database from 2013 to 2017 noted that excluding a single outlying female earner with significant ownership in a company, payments to women were half that of men. The gap widens incredibly when looking at the highest earners. Sullivan and colleagues[11] used the same database to examine the top five highest earning men and women from the 15 highest grossing medical companies from 2013 to 2019. Women were compensated a mean $41,320 versus $1,226,377 for men and, even considering the median, the amount was $20,622 for women versus $129,387 for men ($P < .001$).[11] In the multivariate analysis after accounting for rank, h-index, and specialty the gap between genders still existed with a mean difference of $1,025,413 ($P < .001$).[11] Men had significantly higher industry payments than women across all ranks and specialties.[11]

Potential solutions

- Transparent pay structures based on objective measures, academic rank, or productivity (**Table 1**).
- Remove salary negotiation from compensation models and contracts.
- Implementing university-wide instruction on compensation in accordance with Association of American Medical Colleges western region median salary for rank and specialty led to statistically significant increases in salary for female faculty, and more equality in salary between genders.[12]

Time Allocation at Work

Despite nearly identical number of hours worked per week reported by gender in the AUA 2021 census (53.9 men, 53.8 women), the number of nonclinical hours reported by women was 10.1 versus 8.3 for men, a 20% excess.[1] These nonclinical hours are often filled with such activities as teaching, documenting in the electronic medical record, and/or uncompensated citizenship duties,

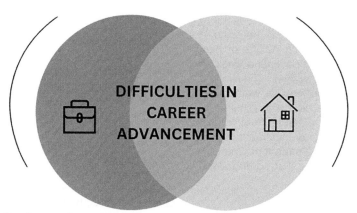

Workplace Issues

- Salary inequity
- Increased time spent on undervalued activities
- Reduced access to research funding
- Unclear promotional criteria
- Fewer leadership and speaking opportunities
- Gendered perceptions of behaviors
- Microaggressions
- Lack of mentorship and sponsorship
- Limited networking opportunities.

Home Issues

- Increased household duties
- Increased parenting duties
- Spouses have competing careers
- Gender bias in the perception of household duties
- Time allocated to maternity leave/lactation

Fig. 1. Difficulties in career advancement for women in urology.

which are less valuable for promotion.[13,14] In a multispecialty high-volume ambulatory center, time spent in the electronic medical record for more than 300 physicians was tracked and women spent 36 minutes greater per week than men, and 41 minutes in the multivariable analysis accounting for patient volume.[15] Additionally, women report spending more time with their patients on average

Table 1 — Active strategies to offset delayed promotion for women in urology	
Women	Ask for promotional criteria in writing, attend seminars Identify mentors a rank up at your institution (may be outside urology) Create a mentorship quilt: people within your society, your section, your faculty who can guide you Have regular discussions with your chairperson regarding trajectory Identify gaps in academic CV early and close them Politely, but firmly set boundaries with support staff
Allies	Correct microaggressions in the workplace to maintain her professional reputation Defend colleagues when standard behavior is labeled aggressive rather than assertive or other gendered stereotypes Engage in work–life balance; normalize time and space for family Sponsorship; offer speaking or leadership opportunities to young women faculty
Institutions	Set a clear standard for what activities do and do not count toward promotion Each subheading (eg, scholarship) needs transparent definitions as to what qualifies and what is important Recognition for mentorship, education, and citizenship duties should be considered Transparent pay structures; consider removing negotiating from salary assignment Provide infrastructure for research to young faculty Provide clinical support so faculty can focus their efforts on career advancement Financial support for coaching and leadership courses Formalized programming to increase awareness and engagement to address gender bias with trackable predefined outcomes and ongoing follow-up

Adapted from Macdonald SM, North AC, "The Gender Gap in Academic Promotion" AUANews April 2024.

(19.3 vs 16.5 minutes per patient).[1] This leads to fewer patient visits per provider, as reflected in the 2021 AUA census in which 42.5% of men report seeing greater than 76 patients a week as compared with only 24% of women.[1] The reasons for these differences are unclear; do women feel compelled to spend more time with patients to be thorough or do patients expect it from women providers? No single activity or increment of time is large, but cumulatively this pattern of time allocation detracts from activities that count toward promotion.

Potential solutions

- Set expectations with staff clearly as to what electronic messages or follow-up is required of urologists and make sure this is applied equally.
- Set an institutional cultural tone that women urologists are equally as busy as their male counterparts and should not have to perform "status leveling" behaviors to be considered part of the team.[16]

Research Funding

Access to research funding is a critical factor in the promotion process at many institutions, and several investigations have identified a gender disparity in access to National Institutes of Health (NIH) funding, which further exacerbates the promotion gap.[17–19] The difficulty in these studies is accounting for differences of experience that would be represented on the biosketch, such as years in practice, research experience, rank, and h-index. In otolaryngology, Eloy and colleagues[18] controlled for academic rank and years of academic practice, yet found that men had significantly higher levels of NIH funding awarded at the assistant professor level and 10 to 20 years of practice. In a study of first time principal investigators applying for NIH grant funding, women received a median of $126,615 as compared with $165,721 for men with a median difference of $39,106 less for women (95% CI, $46,099–$35,675; $P < .001$).[20] Although funding does not directly correlate to productivity or successful research, even small inequities can compound, especially early in a career trajectory.

Potential solutions

- Transparency in the grant award process.
- Support in identifying mentors with similar interest with successful funding histories.
- Diversity among councils or boards reviewing grant applications.

Leadership and Speaking Opportunities

Typically, promotion to associate professor requires a regional reputation and promotion to full professor a nation reputation. Speaking at national meetings, holding leadership positions, or receiving awards by specialty organizations are important ways to demonstrate such a reputation. Multiple studies have shown that major urologic meetings have a significant predominance of all male panels colloquially referred to as "manels."[21,22] Women in the lowest quartile of publications with similar h-indices to their male counterparts, that is, early career urologists, had significantly fewer speaking sessions at major urologic meetings.[22] Similarly, women are mostly awarded lesser type of prestigious AUA awards, such as a presidential citation or young urologist of the year award.[23] Of those given to women 39.5% were given to professionals other than clinical urologists.[23] In looking at the editorial boards of the four highest impact journals in urology between 2000 and 2018, female representation increased, but only from 2.2% to 4.8%, significantly lagging behind proportional representation of the workforce.[24] Additionally, a woman has never held the position of editor-in-chief at a major urologic journal.[24]

Potential solutions

- Intentional consideration of qualified women faculty for leadership and speaking opportunities.
- Develop organizational charts, clearly delineate the selection process for leadership positions, and widely post open positions for greater access to women leaders.
- Implement succession planning that requires transition of positions if preidentified performance goals are not met to encourage turnover and offer more opportunities to women leaders.[25]

WORKPLACE: QUALITATIVE GENDER DISPARITY
Unclear Promotional Criteria

Unclear promotion criteria can cause delays in the promotion process. Ambiguous and opaque criteria can be unevenly applied across different groups, leading to gatekeeping and higher standards for women and minorities to achieve the same ranks. Promotion criteria may not fully acknowledge the contributions of female faculty, because they were established during a time when faculty positions were primarily held by men. Research indicates that women tend to focus more on teaching, mentoring, and service, whereas men tend to prioritize research activities.[26] "Academic productivity" is basically synonymous with research and often the central focus of promotion committees, thus undervaluing other contributions within academia.

Predefined levels of achievement that are explicitly stated to all faculty are critical for fair and equal advancement. In a survey of 567 faculty at a single institution, women physicians were significantly more likely to not receive advisement about promotional criteria (73% vs 58%) and significantly less likely to have a good understanding of promotional criteria (13% vs 26%), compared with their male counterparts.[27] Lack of promotional transparency was the most commonly cited barrier in our prior qualitative study that was designed to assess the relationship of childbirth, parenting, and delayed promotion for women in urology.[28] Multiple participants said they could have been promoted a year earlier had they known from the start more clearly what was expected of them.[28] These findings were confirmed by another qualitative study of 52 women in academic medicine, most of whom were full professors or endowed chairs. In-depth subthemes explored in this study included lack of recognition for clear accomplishments (eg, an R01 grant), "moving the goal post" (requiring further achievement once the predefined level was accomplished), and denial of promotion despite achievement on a level commiserate with or higher than peers.[29] Similarly, in another qualitative assessment of barriers to promotion in general surgery five of nine women (56%) and 2 of 45 men (5%) believed that women were held to a higher standard compared with their male colleagues for promotion.[30] This creates the possibility for biased treatment and the perception of biased treatment to arise, both of which are problematic for career advancement.

Potential solutions

- Self efficacy: Identify resources regarding institutional promotion criteria and set up regular meetings with your supervisor. Identify mentors who have previously gone through the promotions process for support and guidance.
- Transparent promotional criteria: Made available in writing, and in recorded video format, which clearly delineate expectations for each promotional track.
- Directed mentorship programs: Programs targeted to assist with the promotion of women in urology.
- Diversity on promotion and tenure boards: Women in leadership offset implicit or gender bias when reviewing curriculum vitae for promotion.

Citizenship Duties

Citizenship duties refer to activities that are crucial to the mission of the institution, but are not necessarily part of the primary job responsibilities. These duties may include mentoring students, attending nonteaching meetings, and engaging in community service among others. Despite the significant time commitment required of faculty members, these duties are often not considered in promotion criteria. A review found that women were more likely to engage in organizational citizenship behavior related to tasks, yet remain underrecognized compared with their male counterparts.[31] A survey of national women physicians conference attendees found that older women (>49 years of age) and women of color felt obligated to volunteer for citizenship delegations, driven by their age or racial/ethnic background.[32] Despite varying levels of obligation and time commitment, most (67%) female physicians spent about 1 to 5 hours on citizenship duties.[32]

Potential solutions

- Delegate citizenship duties equally within a department.
- Recognition of the time devoted to citizenship duties.

Gendered Perception of Behaviors

The same action or behavior may be perceived differently based on the gender of the individual committing them. In a study of the perception of gender discrimination by academic faculty members women were 2.5 times more likely than men to perceive gender discrimination, whereas women surgeons were 10 times more likely than their male colleagues to perceive gender discrimination.[33] In the 2021 AUA census 66.3% of practicing women urologists reported negative differential treatment based on their gender as compared with 2.7% of men.[32] In particular, fulfilling household duties is frequently seen as a competing demand to work-related responsibilities and may result in doubts about an individual's work ethic and competence. In a qualitative analysis of academic surgeons 31% of men agreed that leaving early or arriving late because of family responsibilities could have an adverse effect on one's career and only 21% believed this was a sign of being a good parent. Conversely, none of the women believed it would be perceived this way.[30] These negative attitudes toward women with household responsibilities can lead to reduced likelihood for promotion or professional recognition.[34] Women face conflicting messages in the workplace, because fulfilling typically female roles is viewed as lacking commitment, whereas adopting masculine traits, such as assertiveness, career-focused ambition, and leadership qualities that demand fair treatment, can trigger a social backlash because it contradicts the expected gender role.

Examples

- A male urologist leaving work early to pick a child up from school might be lauded for his commitment to family, whereas a woman may be perceived as demonstrating a lack of commitment to her career.
- A male urologist who spends less time with a patient might be "busy," whereas a woman might be perceived as "uncaring."
- A male urologist who demands infrastructure for his practice persistently might be seen as assertive or having leadership qualities, whereas a woman might be perceived as demanding, aggressive, or difficult to work with.

These examples and others that result from gendered expectations can negatively impact the working environment, collaborative relationships, and result in less mentorship and sponsorship from senior colleagues.

Potential solutions

- An institutional culture that supports work–life balance of both genders normalizes family obligations outside the workplace.
- Develop cultures within faculty or set by leadership that supports leadership qualities across genders.
- Encourage faculty to identify implicit biases that can impact gender stereotypes. Consider DEI training or implementation of a cultural complications curriculum, which is available by request at https://www.culturalcomplications.com/, to address bias in such areas as identity and advancement and professional development.

Microaggressions

Chester Pierce first coined the term "microaggression" in the 1970s to name the daily slights that African Americans suffered, which constantly remind them of their outsider or "less than" status.[35] This term has been more broadly applied in recent years to all marginalized groups and further subdivided into microinsults, microassaults, and microinvalidations.[36] For women in male-dominated fields, such as urology, microaggressions are constant and unremitting, yet require calm because to be upset would be unprofessional. From the patients, there is the common invalidation that a woman doctor is a nurse or the direct question as to whether she will actually be the surgeon in a case. In a survey of plastic surgery residents 100% of 115 women reported being assumed to be a nurse.[37] These microaggressions no doubt cumulatively contribute to burnout, because in the 2021 AUA census 49% of women reported burnout as compared with 35% in men.[1]

Another common microinsult is the request by support staff to perform small administrative duties that would not be asked of male colleagues. Common examples include calling a patient directly to deliver low acuity results, replacing orders or prescriptions that could be handled by advanced practice providers or nursing staff, prior authorizations, or perhaps even more microassaults/microinvalidations, such as preferentially referring nonsurgical patients (eg, recurrent urinary tract infections) to women urologists. This leads to an unwinnable scenario because to comply with such requests is to delegate time away from those activities that would advance one's career, but to establish boundaries firmly and assert one's self risks behavior incongruous with gender roles that will be perceived as noncollegial, aggressive rather than assertive, and at worst unprofessional. These occurrences also happen in the operating room when women are expected to help clean or transfer the patient, a time when most surgeons dictate or sign in the next patient.[38] These instances represent a trifecta of microaggressions: they invalidate a woman's status compared with her male colleagues by this gendered expectation, they take time away from other activities, and they are a constant source of interpersonal conflict cited in previous studies as a barrier to career advancement.[13,38]

In this paragraph we scratch the surface. Macroaggressions, are sadly not uncommon either and often go unreported because of the concerns regarding anonymity or future career prospects. Although the article is nearly 15 years old, it bears mentioning that in general surgery, a field with significantly more women than urology, in 2004 Schroen and colleagues[39] found that 61% of surveyed female general surgeons experienced sexual harassment, which occurred throughout their career and was perpetrated by physicians (46%), other surgeons (55%), senior surgeons (77%), and patient families (25%).

Potential solutions

- Encouraging open and nonpunitive discussions about professionalism and bias can create an inclusive culture, similar to morbidity and mortality conferences that seek to improve the system rather than condemn errors.

- Institution-wide training on microaggressions as a phenomenon and how to avoid them may be helpful.

Limited Mentorship and Sponsorship

Mentors are those who work alongside mentees and help them attain their desired goals, whereas sponsors are individuals who leverage their position or influence to advocate for an individual typically leading to career advancement. Mentorship and sponsorship have been consistently shown to result in increased clinical productivity, professional development, academic success, and self-confidence in one's career. Having access to mentors and sponsors who can provide advice and guidance on navigating the promotions process is crucial for junior level women to build relationships with senior faculty. Mentors assist women in developing their own networks, and acquiring skills in the various aspects related to academic success, such as grant writing and teaching. Sponsors allow access to opportunities that would otherwise be challenging to achieve, such as national and international speaking, which is necessary for recognition and institutional promotion. Women, however, are consistently noted to have less mentorship compared with their male colleagues.[40] Reasons for this may include the hierarchal nature of medicine, or the pipeline effect with fewer same-sex mentors that can discuss sex-specific issues (pregnancy, motherhood, lactation).[41] Additionally, most mentorships focus on research careers rather than those with a clinical or education focus, both of which are common in women faculty.

Potential solutions

- Intentional sponsorship of women: Suggest women where possible for available leadership, speaking, and collaborative opportunities.
- Develop division/departmental mentorship programs with formalized mentor/mentee training to optimize effectiveness. Obtain institutional funding for support staff and costs associated with programming.

Networking

"The Boys Club" is a colloquial term used to describe networking interactions that take place between men in spaces where women are at least unincluded, and perhaps historically unwelcome. These interactions lead to speaking opportunities, leadership positions, employment, and general advancement in ways that cannot be directly

quantified. In a qualitative assessment of the general surgery faculty at the University of Michigan in 2000, seven women (78%) and nine men (20%) believed women faculty were excluded from informal networking based on gender.[30] In a more recent article in 2021, female plastic surgery trainees also reported feeling excluding from networking and career advancement because of their gender.[37] Less networking may lead to fewer opportunities to collaborate in research or multi-center trials. Caturegli and colleagues[42] noted that women surgeons are less likely to be middle authors as compared with their male colleagues, which may be evidence of this phenomenon.

There is no way to quantify closed door conversations between two parties and how much this is affected by gender and/or ultimately affects a person's career trajectory. That said, the direct corollary to this is women sponsoring women. Talwar and colleagues[43] cataloged speakers at major urologic oncology meetings and found female speakers in sessions were more likely if the chair of the session was also female.

HOME LIFE: GENDER DISPARITY

In the 2021 AUA census 91.7% of practicing urologists report being married.[1] Lerner and colleagues initially reported 67% of women having biologic children in 2009 and in the updated data published by Scott and Lerner in 2020, 78% of women queried reported biologic children.[44,45] An additional 12 of the 167 women (7%) surveyed reported step-children or an adopted child. Although not all women are married or have children at home, certainly these data show that most have children and a spouse.

Differences in the Burden of Household Duties

It has been observed that household chores and parenting duties are primarily shouldered by women, which often poses an obstacle to engaging in promotion-generating activities. In AUA census data from 2018, 20% of women respondents were primarily responsible for household duties, whereas only 25% had partners who were primarily responsible as compared with a stark 8% of men who were primarily responsible for household duties and almost half or 49% of partners of male urologists who were primarily responsible for household duties.[5] A 2009 survey study of 895 American Board of Surgery certified surgeons reported that 80% of women had a spouse with a career, whereas only 40% of men reported the same.[46] Furthermore, 56.3% of men reported a homemaker spouse, whereas only 9.4% of women surgeons had the same level of support at home.[46] In a study of 54 faculty surgeons at the University of Michigan regarding perceived barriers to academic advancement women were significantly more likely to miss work because of family responsibilities 56% (women) versus 20% (men), whereas men were more likely to miss family events because of job demands 77% (men) versus 67% (women).[30] Nearly all respondents were married with children; however, the mean number of parenting duties and household chores for men per week was 17.6 and 8 hours, respectively, whereas women reported 33.8 and 10.9 hours, a staggeringly high figure.[30] It is uncertain whether this disparity is caused by traditional gender roles or by the fact that all female faculty members reported having a working spouse, whereas only 33% of male faculty members reported having a part-time working spouse and another 36% reported having a spouse who stays at home. Having a spouse with a less demanding career, who works from home, or does not work enables the surgeon spouse to focus their time and effort on career-oriented activities. Unsurprisingly, spousal support was cited as a major advantage toward academic promotion in our recent qualitative review of women in academic urology.[28]

Potential solutions

- Onsite daycare.
- Ability to participate in early morning and late afternoon meetings remotely.
- Flexible work schedules to accommodate those with career spouses or children.

Maternity Leave and Lactation

According to the 2019 census 90.6% of practicing urologists report having children.[47] In a survey of 243 board-certified women urologists reported in 2009, Lerner and colleagues[44] noted that the average age of birth of a first child was 32.6, for a second child 35.1, and for a third child 36.5. In an update to these data surveying 186 board-certified women urologists, Scott and Lerner[45] compared women who graduated before and after 2007 and showed an increase in the number of women choosing to have their first child during residency as opposed to fellowship or practice. On average more than 40% have their first child in practice and nearly 60% for a second child; this timing aligns with early career as an assistant professor given that the average time it takes to progress to assistant has been reported as 6 years.[45,48] On average the cohort in Scott and Lerner[45] reported two children with most taking between 5 and 12 weeks of leave; thus on average 2 to 6 months of academic practice are missed by women in their early career. This is not to mention

the challenges of mental acuity and academic productivity on returning to work postpartum, which was cited in a qualitative study on barriers to promotion for women in urology.[28] Last, the sheer time allocated to lactation by 6 months of exclusive breastfeeding as recommended by the American Academy of Pediatrics is counter to clinical and academic productivity.[49]

SUMMARY

There is a saying "you cannot fight a battle on all fronts," and essentially that is what women do. They fight implicit gender bias, quantifiably lower funding and salary, higher standards, and increased time demands because of gender roles at home and at work. As Bickel[50] described the phenomenon, cumulative career disadvantages, it is a losing battle when one fights on all fronts and promotion is delayed.

The attempts to mitigate these gender disparities are as controversial as the disparities themselves. No woman wants to feel as though she is a token speaker on a panel selected solely for her gender. No man wants to feel slighted because someone filled a diversity quota. The most palatable first steps would be to implement programs that are egalitarian, that benefit all members of the workforce. Transparent pay structures, transparent promotional criteria, support for parental leave, and flexible work schedules that support faculty with young children would be helpful for all genders and those with minority status. Next, dedicated leadership and formalized mentorship programs for women within surgical subspecialties are needed to help actively combat the obstacles presented within this article. Finally, as more women in urology rise to senior status and leadership positions, individual women with strong voices and positions of power will likely be instrumental in highlighting and correcting continued disparities.

CLINICS CARE POINTS

- Active strategies to close the gender gap in promotions are necessary including mentorship programs, transparent promotional criteria and pay, equitable research funding, as well as opportunities for leadership and speaking for women.

- Institutional programs are needed to help individuals identify their own implicit bias and address it to assuage differences in the perception of professionalism and prevent microaggressions from occuring.

DISCLOSURE

S.M. MacDonald has the following disclosures: Boston Scientific, consultant; VidScrip, consultant and research funding. R.D. Malik has the following disclosures: Urovant Sciences, speaker.

REFERENCES

1. The State of the Urology Workforce and Practice in the United States 2021. Available at: https://www.auanet.org/documents/research/census/2021%20Census%20Report.pdf, Accessed: March 2023.

2. Awad MA, Gaither TW, Osterberg EC, et al. Gender differences in promotions and scholarly productivity in academic urology. Can J Urol 2017;24:9011–6.

3. Breyer BN, Butler C, Fang R, et al. Promotion disparities in academic urology. Urology 2020;138:16–23.

4. Richter KP, Clark L. Women physicians and promotion in academic medicine. N Engl J Med 2020; 383:2148–57.

5. The State of the Urology Workforce and Practice in the United States 2018. Available at: https://www.auanet.org/documents/research/census/2018%20The%20State%20of%20the%20Urology%20Workforce%20Census%20Book.pdf, Accessed: March 2023.

6. Bradbury CL, King DK, Middleton RG. Female urologists: a growing population. J Urol 1997;157: 1854–6.

7. Lightner DJ, Terris MK, Tsao AK, et al. Status of women in urology: based on a report to the Society of University Urologists. J Urol 2005;173:560–3.

8. Spencer ES, Deal AM, Pruthi NR, et al. Gender differences in compensation, job satisfaction and other practice patterns in urology. J Urol 2016;195:450–5.

9. North AC, Fang R, Anger J, et al. The gender pay gap in urology. Urology Practice 2021;8:149–54.

10. Velez D, Mehta A, Rotker K, et al. Gender disparities in industry payments to urologists. Urology 2021; 150:59–64.

11. Sullivan BG, Al-Khouja F, Herre M, et al. Assessment of medical industry compensation to US physicians by gender. JAMA Surg 2022;157:1017–22.

12. Hoops HE, Brasel KJ, Dewey E, et al. Analysis of gender-based differences in surgery faculty compensation, promotion, and retention: establishing equity. Ann Surg 2018;268:479–87.

13. Thompson-Burdine JA, Telem DA, Waljee JF, et al. Defining barriers and facilitators to advancement for women in academic surgery. JAMA Netw Open 2019;2:e1910228.

14. Armijo PR, Silver JK, Larson AR, et al. Citizenship tasks and women physicians: additional woman tax in academic medicine? J Womens Health (Larchmt) 2021;30:935–43.

15. Rotenstein LS, Fong AS, Jeffery MM, et al. Gender differences in time spent on documentation and the electronic health record in a large ambulatory network. JAMA Netw Open 2022;5:e223935.

16. Cardador MT, Hill PL, Salles A. Unpacking the status-leveling burden for women in male-dominated occupations. Adm Sci Q 2021;67: 237–84.

17. Berg EJ, Ashurst J. Patterns of recent National Institutes of Health (NIH) funding in general surgery: analysis using the NIH RePORTER system. Cureus 2019;11:e4938.

18. Eloy JA, Svider PF, Kovalerchik O, et al. Gender differences in successful NIH grant funding in otolaryngology. Otolaryngol Head Neck Surg 2013;149: 77–83.

19. Franceschi AM, Rosenkrantz AB. Patterns of recent National Institutes of Health (NIH) funding to diagnostic radiology departments: analysis using the NIH RePORTER System. Acad Radiol 2017;24: 1162–8.

20. Oliveira DFM, Ma Y, Woodruff TK, et al. Comparison of National Institutes of Health grant amounts to first-time male and female principal investigators. JAMA 2019;321:898–900.

21. Harris KT, Clifton MM, Matlaga BR, et al. Gender representation among plenary panel speakers at the American Urological Association annual meeting. Urology 2021;150:54–8.

22. Teoh JY, Castellani D, Mercader C, et al. A quantitative analysis investigating the prevalence of "manels" in major urology meetings. Eur Urol 2021;80:442–9.

23. Wenzel J, Dudley A, Agnor R, et al. Women are underrepresented in prestigious recognition awards in the American Urological Association. Urology 2022; 160:102–8.

24. Henderson AA, Murray KS, Ahmed H. Female representation on journal editorial boards: is urology behind the times? J Urol 2019;201:237–8.

25. Identifying gender disparities and barriers to measuring the status of female faculty: the experience of a large school of medicine. J Wom Health 2019;28:1569–75.

26. Misra J, Lundquist JH, Templer A. Gender, work time, and care responsibilities among faculty 1. In: Sociological Forum27. Oxford, UK: Blackwell Publishing Ltd.; 2012. p. 300–23.

27. Buckley LM, Sanders K, Shih M, et al. Obstacles to promotion? Values of women faculty about career success and recognition. Acad Med 2000; 75:283–8.

28. MacDonald SM, Malik RD. Women in academic urology: a qualitative analysis of the relationship between pregnancy, parenting, and delayed promotion. Urology 2022;168:13–20.

29. Murphy M, Callander JK, Dohan D, et al. Women's experiences of promotion and tenure in academic medicine and potential implications for gender

disparities in career advancement: a qualitative analysis. JAMA Netw Open 2021;4:e2125843.

30. Colletti LM, Mulholland MW, Sonnad SS. Perceived obstacles to career success for women in academic surgery. Arch Surg 2000;135:972–7.

31. Ng TWH, Lam SSK, Feldman DC. Organizational citizenship behavior and counterproductive work behavior: do males and females differ? J Vocat Behav 2016;93:11–32.

32. Citizenship tasks and women physicians: additional woman tax in academic medicine? J Wom Health 2021;30:935–43.

33. Carr PL, Ash AS, Friedman RH, et al. Faculty perceptions of gender discrimination and sexual harassment in academic medicine. Ann Intern Med 2000;132:889–96.

34. Gender discrimination in the medical profession. Council on Ethical and Judicial Affairs. American Medical Association. Wom Health Issues 1994;4:1–11.

35. Pierce CM. Black psychiatry one year after Miami. J Natl Med Assoc 1970;62:471–3.

36. Torres MB, Salles A, Cochran A. Recognizing and reacting to microaggressions in medicine and surgery. JAMA Surg 2019;154:868–72.

37. Chen W, Schilling BK, Bourne DA, et al. A report of gender bias and sexual harassment in current plastic surgery training: a national survey. Plast Reconstr Surg 2021;147:1454–68.

38. Cardador MT, Hill PL, Salles A. Unpacking the status-leveling burden for women in male-dominated occupations. Adm Sci Q 2022;67:237–84.

39. Schroen AT, Brownstein MR, Sheldon GF. Women in academic general surgery. Acad Med 2004;79(4):310–8.

40. The State of Women in Academic Medicine. Available at: https://www.aamc.org/data-reports/data/2018-2019-state-women-academic-medicine-exploring-pathways-equity, Accessed: March.

41. Murphy AM, Shenot PJ, Lallas CD. Faculty development: how do we encourage faculty to become better teachers and mentors? Curr Urol Rep 2020;21:40.

42. Caturegli I, Caturegli G, Hays N, et al. Trends in female surgeon authorship: the role of the middle author. Am J Surg 2020;220:1541–8.

43. Talwar R, Bernstein A, Jones A, et al. Assessing contemporary trends in female speakership within urologic oncology. Urology 2021;150:41–6.

44. Lerner LB, Stolzmann KL, Gulla VD. Birth trends and pregnancy complications among women urologists. J Am Coll Surg 2009;208:293–7.

45. Scott VCS, Lerner LB. Re-evaluation of birth trends and pregnancy complications among female urologists: have we made any progress? Neurourol Urodyn 2020;39:1355–62.

46. Troppmann KM, Palis BE, Goodnight JE Jr, et al. Women surgeons in the new millennium. Arch Surg 2009;144:635–42.

47. The State of Urology Workforce and Practice in the United States 2019. Available at: https://www.auanet.org/documents/research/census/2019-State-of-Urology-Workforce-Census-Book.pdf, Accessed: March 2023.

48. Liu C.Q.A.H., Promotion rates for first-time assistant and associate professors appointed from 1967 to 1997, 9(7), *AAMC Analysis in Brief*, 2010, 1-2.

49. Amercian Academy of Pediatrics Breast Feeding Recommendations. Available at: https://publications.aap.org/aapnews/news/20528/Updated-AAP-guidance-recommends-longer?autologincheck=redirected, Accessed: March 2023.

50. Bickel J. Maximizing professional development of women in medicine. The Scientist; 1997. Available at: https://www.the-scientist.com/commentary/maximizing-professional-development-of-women-in-academic-medicine-57487. Accessed: March 2023.

The Other Pandemic, Racism, in Urology

Olutiwa Akinsola, MD, MS[a],*, Adam P. Klausner, MD[b], Randy Vince, MD[c], Kristen R. Scarpato, MD[a]

KEYWORDS

- Diversity • Racism • Pipeline • Pandemic

KEY POINTS

- Structural racism continues to impact patient care, education, and research within medicine, and the field of Urology is not immune from its effects.
- Minority patients have been shown to have delayed or subpar treatment compared with their white counterparts.
- There remains a paucity of underrepresented patient participation in urologic clinical trials, likely owing to longstanding mistrust of the scientific community because of abuses of the past.
- Many initiatives have been put in place to increase diversity in Urology, including pipeline programs, creating more holistic residency application review, and seeking more diverse voices within research publications.

Racism is deeply ingrained in our society, and medicine has not been immune to this bias. The recent COVID-19 pandemic further highlighted racial disparities in the medical field. Injustice and discrimination also exist in the field of Urology, prompting investigation into the effects on education and patient care. This article reviews the current literature regarding structural racism in medicine and urology, the "other pandemic," and provides recommendations for focused efforts to eliminate systemic racial inequities.

Racism is the belief that some races or ethnicities are superior to others, and this idea is used to justify actions that create inequality.[1] Racism is not always obvious and has evolved in many instances into a more subtle and covert expression of prejudice.[2] These divisive beliefs persist in health care; despite overall increased life expectancy in the United States, minority populations continue to have higher rates of morbidity and mortality compared with white persons.[3] Studies demonstrate that minority patients receive lower-quality care and fewer procedures compared with their white counterparts.[4]

More recently, racial disparities in surgery have become a regular topic of robust discussion. Multiple studies have shown that black patients have higher rates of mortality following major operations, including carotid endarterectomy, aortic valve replacement, cystectomy, abdominal aortic aneurysm repair, resection of lung cancer, coronary artery bypass graft, and pancreatic resection.[5] These disparate outcomes are likely due to racial differences in screening, diagnosis, patient counseling, and treatment. This was highlighted by Morris and colleagues,[6] who found that for patients with colorectal cancer, black people were diagnosed at younger ages but with more advanced disease, and treatment modalities differed significantly between races. Similar

Note: race/ethnicity denotes that both race and ethnicity were combined in this analysis, but that race and ethnicity are distinctly different and not synonymous.

[a] Department of Urology, Vanderbilt University Medical Center, 1211 Medical Center Drive, Nashville, TN 37232, USA; [b] Division of Urology, Department of Surgery, Virginia Commonwealth University School of Medicine, 1200 East Broad Street, 7th Floor East Wing, Richmond, VA 23298, USA; [c] Case Western Reserve University, University Hospital Urology Institute, 11100 Euclid Avenue, Cleveland, OH 44106, USA
* Corresponding author.
E-mail address: Olutiwa.akinsola@vumc.org

Urol Clin N Am 50 (2023) 525–530
https://doi.org/10.1016/j.ucl.2023.06.012
0094-0143/23/Published by Elsevier Inc.

findings were also noted in women with endometrial cancer—black women were significantly less likely to undergo surgery with shorter survival times in comparison to white women.[7]

With continued and increasing evidence of racial disparities in medicine and surgery, calls for mitigating these inequities have been seen on the federal level. In 2011, the largest federal-based plan of action to reduce health care inequities was put forth by the US Department of Health and Human Services.[8] This plan provided incentives aimed at increasing quality health care for minority patients while building a database of the care provided while assessing improvements in disparities over time.[8] Best and colleagues[9] highlighted this initiative as a time stamp to determine if there were any improvements in surgical disparities following implementation and, unfortunately, found that disparities persisted in all of the procedures analyzed after its initiation. Another study evaluated cancer-related surgery mortality from 2007 to 2016, finding that although mortalities declined overall, there was a persistent gap between races with black patients having a higher mortality than whites.[10] The accumulated evidence confirms that within surgery, racial disparities continue to exist in care delivery, which significantly impacts patient outcomes.

The surgical subspecialty of urology also suffers from racism and its far-reaching negative consequences. Data indicate that racial inequities adversely impact multiple aspects of patient care and outcomes. For men with prostate cancer, this disparity exists across the continuum of care, from screening practices to patient counseling and recommended treatments. One study evaluating the rates of prostate cancer screening showed that black and Hispanic men had lower rates of prostate cancer screening even when adjusting for access to care, smoking, and age.[11] Underwood and colleagues[12] found that black and Hispanic men with clinically significant prostate cancer were less likely to receive definitive treatment when compared with white men. Another study found that in black men and white men with similar prostate cancer disease characteristics, black men were more likely to receive nonsurgical management.[13] Studies looking at treatment decisional regret in patients with prostate cancer found that black and non-white men were more likely to experience regret following prostate cancer treatment in comparison to white men.[14–16] This supports the notion that minority men with prostate cancer may be receiving subpar pretreatment counseling compared with their white counterparts. Acknowledging these disparate outcomes, one study evaluated the potential benefit of decision aids to improve knowledge for prostate cancer treatment in a diverse patient population, but unfortunately, did not demonstrate meaningful gains in prostate cancer knowledge.[17]

These findings are not limited to prostate cancer. Within Pediatric Urology, Ahn and colleagues[18] found that Hispanic and black boys with cryptorchidism had significant delays to orchiopexy in comparison to white boys; black boys were delayed by 7 months, whereas Hispanic boys were delayed by 5 months after adjusting for developmental delays and comorbidities. For patients with muscle-invasive bladder cancer, racial differences in rates of guideline-based treatment have been found, with one study showing black patients had a 21% lower odds of receiving treatment recommended by organizational guidelines in comparison to white patients.[19] Another study showed black patients have a higher rate of 90-day mortality when compared with white counterparts.[20]

Racial disparity permeates research as well. There is a well-established lack of diversity within recruitment for clinical trials. Woods-Burnham and colleagues[21] reported that one-third of clinical trials that lead to cancer drug approval did not report on the races/ethnicities of the participants. Within bladder and kidney cancer clinical trials, Javier-DesLoges and colleagues[22] found that black and Hispanic patients were underrepresented compared with white patients. Interestingly, when looking at black participation from 2000 to 2019, the investigators found that rates were stagnant—no progress had been made in the recruitment of black patients over nearly 2 decades. In a study evaluating black participation in genitourinary clinical trials that led to novel drug approval between 2015 and 2020, results indicated that enrollment in prostate cancer trials declined and was unchanged for trials assessing urothelial carcinoma.[23] One major cause for disparities within clinical research is the history of victimization of minority groups by the medical community via unethical experimentation. The Tuskegee Syphilis study, the cells harvested from Henrietta Lacks without consent, and the illegal sterilization of thousands of Native American women during the 1970s are just a few examples of inappropriate medical experimentation within underrepresented populations. This unjust history within medical research remains a barrier to the enrollment of many minority patients in clinical trials. The medical and research community must work to regain the trust of minority patients so that our field can achieve inclusive and effective treatments for all populations.

This lack of diversity within clinical trials has also been observed in medical publishing in Urology. The editorial titled "We've Got a Long Way to Go, and a Short Time to Get There" highlighted that increasing diversity within leadership of the *Journal of Urology* can help to bring varied experiences, opinions, and insight into the literature published within the field.[24] The author appropriately noted that one cause of limited diversity in medical publishing is the low number of minority providers currently holding academic positions in Urology; this underscores the fact that improvements in the urology pipeline can have far-reaching effects for the field, including diversity in the realm of scientific publication.

The impact of racism is also evident within the urologic training community. The current workforce does not reflect the population it serves, in part due to the "leaky pipeline." American Urological Association (AUA) Census data indicate that only about 2% of practicing urologists are black/African American, a number that has been stagnant for many years, and about 5% self-identify as Latinx/Hispanic.[25] Across US urology training programs, about 3.5% and 4% of residents are black/African American and Latinx/Hispanic, respectively.[26] Underrepresented in medicine (URiM) applicants to urology lag in comparison to the national population. Successful recruitment of minority applicants into urology residency is necessary for improving diversity in our field. At the residency program level, review committees at many institutions have adopted a more holistic application review process, conducted virtual interviews to level the playing field and limit costs, and offered scholarships for diverse students to pursue away electives. These efforts are important but represent only one aspect where more work is needed. Future aims should focus on interventions that foster improved diversity at every step of the educational pipeline.

Fortunately, within urology, there are many current efforts underway to improve diversity within the field, including addressing the pipeline. The R. Frank Jones Society was formed in 1965 and named after Dr Jones, who was the first black urologist certified by the American Board of Urology in 1936. In an effort to combat health care disparity, the Society mentors and sponsors black students who endeavor to become urologists while continuously advocating for equitable policies and appropriate resources to build the pipeline. Their goals include increasing the number of black urologists, reducing health care barriers for black patients in clinical trial enrollment, and promoting race-concordant care for improved patient outcomes.[27]

Also addressing the pipeline, the Mid-Atlantic section of the AUA now offers a Pre-Medicine Enrichment Program aimed at "empowering historically underrepresented minorities who are first-generation students considering medicine" (https://maaua.org/pep/). The 8-week program focuses on mentorship and clinical research while offering a comprehensive opportunity to shadow across clinical settings, including the office and operating room. Commonly, students are undergraduate sophomores or juniors who continue to check in with mentors annually following the program for long-term, meaningful career development.

The recently initiated AUA Diversity Equity and Inclusion (DEI) Committee currently comprises 13 urologists who have knowledge, experience, and passion for supporting and sponsoring marginalized patients and providers within Urology. In its short existence, this committee has undertaken several important endeavors, including launching the podcast series titled *AUANews Inside Tract Podcast, Voices* where committee members and invited special guests discuss important topics within DEI, including mentorship and increasing the number of providers working in this space. More recently, the committee contacted training programs with the goal of helping to foster diversity in the community of educators and residents. Through surveying Urology Residency Program Directors, they hope to determine ongoing residency program efforts to support underrepresented students in medicine. Ultimately, this effort will result in curation of a list of Visiting Student Learning Opportunities that includes scholarships directed at students URiM, a much-needed step for improved diversity among urology training programs.[28]

Urology Unbound is another group aimed at increasing representation of URiM within Urology. The program's vision is to build a urology workforce that mirrors the diversity of the communities served in an effort to erase urologic health disparities. It was formed by black fellows and early-career faculty members during the COVID-19 pandemic to help black and brown applicants navigate the application and virtual interview process for Urology residency. They offer not only resident application review and mock virtual interviews but also networking opportunities and mentorship at each level of training.[29]

At the University of Michigan, the Department of Urology created the Michigan Urology Academy (MUA) in 2020 with the goal of increasing diversity in the urologic workforce by improving opportunity and access for all. Through multiple virtual workshops aimed at future urology applicants, underrepresented faculty from institutions across the nation have been able to share their personal experiences and provide direct mentorship. Workshops have offered advice for success on the urology subinternship and strategies for managing microaggressions in the workplace. This year, MUA is planning an in-person, all-expenses-paid event for minority students without a home urology program where participants will interact with current residents and prepare their residency applications.[30]

Another group formed to address the lack of diversity within urology during the COVID-19 pandemic is the UReTER (UnderRepresented Trainees Entering Residency) Mentorship Program. It was formed in June 2020 by the urology residents at the University of California San Francisco. Through this mentorship model, urology residents are paired with medical students who identify as black, indigenous, Native Hawaiian, and/or Latinx to guide these medical students through the application and interview process on the path to successful residency match. Participants' response to this mentorship program has been subsequently evaluated, and the program was found to be feasible, acceptable to both mentors and mentees, and most notably increased mentees' chances of a successful Urology match.[31]

Individual efforts within the field have also been initiated to better understand factors that positively or negatively impact equity, diversity, and inclusion in urology residency. Recently, an anonymous survey was distributed to urology residents nationally directly querying trainees on influential aspects encountered in the pipeline to urology. Similarly, many individual medical schools have implemented mandatory surgical subspecialty rotations, improving the visibility of Urology to medical students.

The efforts to improve diversity have also begun at the provider level within urologic academia. In an editorial titled "Reflections on Diversity, Equity and Inclusion in Medical Publishing: The Journal of Urology HEAD table," the authors highlighted the lack of diversity within the scientific leadership community and proposed that increasing representation of underrepresented scientists in the field can help combat this issue. Motivated board members within the *Journal of Urology* organized to create a space for discussions related to health equity and diversity called the HEAD table. They endeavor to successfully increase diversity within their publications board from others in the scientific community by holding a regular diversity, equity, and inclusion Webinar series. This spurred the idea of the first open call for editorial positions within the *Journal of Urology*, which attracted

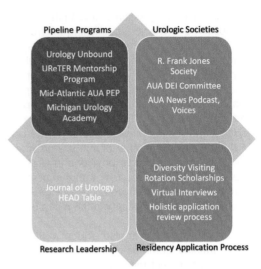

Fig. 1. Different initiatives within urology aimed at addressing diversity, equity, and inclusion.

several strong and diverse applicants, and the Journal plans to continue this practice moving forward.[32] All of the above initiatives are included in **Fig. 1**.

It remains abundantly clear that racism persists in medicine, including within the field of Urology. The broad scope of the problem has been well-described and demonstrated repeatedly. Also readily apparent and well-enumerated are the many benefits of diversity in the workforce. Nevertheless, there are ongoing initiatives to thwart any forward progress addressing racial disparities, including recent action to remove DEI programs from some individual state institutions. Medicine must take action to fix these problems if the field is to eliminate disparity and improve health care outcomes across all populations. Currently, many efforts are underway, but this "other pandemic" persists.

CLINICS CARE POINTS

- Within the field of Urology, the effects of racism impact many aspects of patient care leading to poorer outcomes for minority patients.

- Pipeline programs focused on medical students interested in Urology can help to improve diversity within the workforce.

- Increasing diversity within urologic academia requires intentional initiatives that create more space for those underrepresented in medicine.

DISCLOSURE

The authors have nothing to disclose.

REFERENCES

1. Bhopal R. Racism in medicine. BMJ 2001; 322(7301):1503–4.
2. Bonilla-Silva E. *Racism without racists: color-blind racism and the persistence of racial inequality in America.* 3. Lanham: Rowman & Littlefield Publishers; 2009. p. 318.
3. Williams DR, Rucker TD. Understanding and addressing racial disparities in health care. Health Care Financ Rev 2000;21(4):75–90.
4. Williams DR, Wyatt R. Racial bias in health care and health: challenges and opportunities. JAMA 2015; 314(6):555–6 [Erratum in: JAMA. 2015 Sep 15; 314(11):1179. PMID: 26262792].
5. Lucas FL, Stukel TA, Morris AM, et al. Race and surgical mortality in the United States. Ann Surg 2006; 243(2):281–6.
6. Morris AM, Billingsley KG, Baxter NN, et al. Racial disparities in rectal cancer treatment: a population-based analysis. Arch Surg 2004;139(2):151–5 [discussion: 156].
7. Randall TC, Armstrong K. Differences in treatment and outcome between African-American and white women with endometrial cancer. J Clin Oncol 2003;21(22):4200–6.
8. US Department of Health and Human Services . HHS action plan to reduce racial and ethnic disparities: a nation free of disparities in health and health care. Published April 2011. Available at: https://www.minorityhealth.hhs.gov/npa/files/Plans/HHS/HHS_Plan_complete.pdf. Accessed June 15, 2020.
9. Best MJ, McFarland EG, Thakkar SC, et al. Racial disparities in the use of surgical procedures in the US. JAMA Surg 2021;156(3):274–81.
10. Lam MB, Raphael K, Mehtsun WT, et al. Changes in racial disparities in mortality after cancer surgery in the US, 2007-2016. JAMA Netw Open 2020;3(12): e2027415.
11. Riviere P, Kalavacherla S, Banegas MP, et al. Patient perspectives of prostate cancer screening vary by race following 2018 guideline changes. Cancer 2023;129(1):82–8.
12. Underwood W, De Monner S, Ubel P, et al. Racial/ethnic disparities in the treatment of localized/regional prostate cancer. J Urol 2004;171(4):1504–7.
13. Moses KA, Paciorek AT, Penson DF, et al. Impact of ethnicity on primary treatment choice and mortality in men with prostate cancer: data from CaPSURE. J Clin Oncol 2010;28(6):1069–74.
14. Hu JC, Kwan L, Krupski TL, et al. Determinants of treatment regret in low-income, uninsured men with prostate cancer. Urology 2008;72(6): 1274–9.
15. Schroeck FR, Krupski TL, Sun L, et al. Satisfaction and regret after open retropubic or robot-assisted laparoscopic radical prostatectomy. Eur Urol 2008;54(4):785–93. Epub 2008 Jun 23. PMID: 18585849.
16. Morris BB, Farnan L, Song L, et al. Treatment decisional regret among men with prostate cancer: Racial differences and influential factors in the North Carolina Health Access and Prostate Cancer Treatment Project (HCaP-NC). Cancer 2015; 121(12):2029–35. Epub 2015 Mar 3. PMID: 25740564.
17. Tilburt JC, Zahrieh D, Pacyna JE, et al. Decision aids for localized prostate cancer in diverse minority men: primary outcome results from a multicenter cancer care delivery trial (Alliance A191402CD). Cancer 2022;128(6):1242–51.
18. Ahn JJ, Garrison MM, Merguerian PA, et al. Racial and ethnic disparities in the timing of orchiopexy for cryptorchidism. J Pediatr Urol 2022 Oct;18(5): 696.e1–6. Epub 2022 Sep 11. PMID: 36175288; PMCID: PMC9771941.
19. Washington SL 3rd, Gregorich SE, Meng MV, et al. Race modifies survival benefit of guideline-based treatment: Implications for reducing disparities in muscle invasive bladder cancer. Cancer Med 2020;9(22):8310–7. Epub 2020 Sep 1. PMID: 32869516; PMCID: PMC7666728.
20. Marinaro J, Zeymo A, Egan J, et al. Sex and racial disparities in the treatment and outcomes of muscle-invasive bladder cancer. Urology 2021;151: 154–62. Epub 2020 Aug 15. PMID: 32810481.
21. Woods-Burnham L, Johnson JR, Hooker SE Jr, et al. The role of diverse populations in US clinical trials. Med (New York, N.Y.) 2021;2(1):21–4.
22. Javier-DesLoges J, Nelson TJ, Murphy JD, et al. An evaluation of trends in the representation of patients by age, sex, and diverse race/ethnic groups in bladder and kidney cancer clinical trials. Urol Oncol 2022;40(5):199.e15–21.
23. Matthew-Onabanjo AN, Nortey G, Matulewicz RS, et al. Diversity, equity, and inclusion in genitourinary clinical trials leading to FDA novel drug approval: An assessment of the FDA center for drug evaluation and research drug trials snapshot. Curr Probl Cancer 2023;47(3):100958. Advance online publication.
24. Siemens DR. We've got a long way to go, and a short time to get there. J Urol 2022;208(1):4–5.
25. AUA. AUA Annual Census 2020. AUA. Available at: https://www.auanet.org/research-and-data/aua-census/census-results. Accessed June 7, 2023.
26. Simons ECG, Arevalo A, Samuel L, et al. Trends in the Racial and Ethnic Diversity in the US Urology Workforce. Urology 2022;162:9–19.

27. Guest. (2023, May 23). Promoting diversity and empowering black urologists: The R. frank jones urological society - Linda L. McIntire. UroToday. Available at: https://www.urotoday.com/video-lectures/aua-2023/video/3406-promoting-diversity-and-empowering-black-urologists-the-r-frank-jones-urological-society-linda-l-mcintire.html. Accessed June 5, 2023.

28. Diversity, Equity and Inclusion. Diversity, equity and Inclusion - American Urological Association. (2023). Available at: https://www.auanet.org/diversity-equity-and-inclusion. Accessed June 5, 2023.

29. Our story. Urology Unbound - Our Story. (2022). Available at: https://urologyunbound.org/Our-Story. Accessed June 4, 2023.

30. Michigan Urology Academy (mua): Urology: Michigan medicine. Urology. (2023, June 5). Available at: https://medicine.umich.edu/dept/urology/education/medical-students/michigan-urology-academy-mua. Accessed June 5, 2023.

31. Zheng MY, Overland M, Escobar D, et al. Formal mentorship as an opportunity to expand the urology pipeline: under represented trainees entering residency (UReTER) program evaluation 2020-2021. Urology 2022;162:108–13.

32. Avulova S, Enemchukwu E, Kaufman M, et al. Reflections on diversity, equity, and inclusion in medical publishing: *The Journal of Urology* HEAD Table. J Urol 2023;209(5):830–2.

Linguistic Differences Based on Gender and Race in Urology Application Personal Statements
A Comparison of 2017 and 2023 Applications

Emma C. Bethel, MD[a,1], Asia N. Matthew-Onabanjo, MD, PhD[a,1],
Hannah E. Kay, MD[a], Ram Basak, PhD[a], Alysen Demzik, MD[a],
Pauline Filippou, MD[b], Davis Viprakasit, MD[a], Kristy M. Borawski, MD[a],
Eric M. Wallen, MD[a], Angela B. Smith, MD, MS[a],
Hung-Jui Tan, MD, MSHPM[a,*]

KEYWORDS

- Diversity • Equity • Inclusion • Linguistics • Urology/education • Internship and residency • Gender
- Race

KEY POINTS

- Modest linguistic differences in personal statements exist for female and URM applicants to urology compared to their male and NHW counterparts, respectively.
- Difference in linguistic qualities by gender and race have not changed substantively over time despite increased Diversity and Inclusion efforts in urology.
- The linguistic differences for URMs may be vulnerable to ongoing biases that negatively impact entrance into urology.

INTRODUCTION

Despite efforts to increase diversity across medical fields, women and certain minorities remain underrepresented in urology. The 2022 American Urologic Association (AUA) Census shows that while there has been a significant increase in the number of practicing female urologists over the last 4 decades, women still represent only 11.6% of the urologic workforce.[1] Furthermore, according to United States census data, 13.6% of the US population identifies as Black/African American while 18.9%

identify as Hispanic or Latino.[2] In contrast, only 2.2% and 4.9% of current practicing urologists identify as Black/African American or Latinx/Hispanic, respectively.[1] Unlike workforce trends observed for women, the percent of Black/African American trainees (5.2%) and Latinx/Hispanic trainees (8.4%) have remained low and slower to increase despite more recent efforts for recruitment and retention.[3–5]

The lack of diversity in urology has been well-recognized by the AUA and the Society of

Note: race/ethnicity–denotes that both race and ethnicity were combined in this analysis, but that race and ethnicity are distinctly different and not synonymous.

[a] Department of Urology, School of Medicine, University of North Carolina, Chapel Hill, NC, USA;
[b] Department of Urology, Kaiser Permanente Northern California, Santa Clara Medical Center, Santa Clara, CA, USA
[1] co-first authors.
* Corresponding author. Department of Urology, University of North Carolina, Chapel Hill, 2116 Physician Office Building, Campus Box 7235, Chapel Hill, NC 27599-7235.
E-mail address: ray_tan@med.unc.edu

Urol Clin N Am 50 (2023) 531–539
https://doi.org/10.1016/j.ucl.2023.06.013

Academic Urologists (SAU). To foster a more inclusive workforce environment and address disparities in urologic care, the AUA created a diversity and inclusion task force in 2020, and the SAU created a similar task force whose goal is to recruit and retain women and minority urologists.[6–9] While the definition of URM can vary, this categorization generally includes those who identify as Black, Latinx/Hispanic or of Spanish origin, Native American, Native Alaskan, and Pacific Islander; all groups that are not represented in the medical field to the same degree they are in the general population. Multiple urology programs have made an active effort to acknowledge this gap and create fully funded visiting acting internships (AIs) for underrepresented groups to improve gender and racial diversity at their programs.[10–13] However, it remains unclear whether these efforts to promote diversity and inclusion have resulted in tangible differences in the way women and URMs are mentored, supported, and recruited into urology. Previously, we analyzed personal statements from urology residency applications from the 2016-2017 cycle, which showed modest linguistic differences by gender and race/ethnicity. In that cycle, males used words that indicated acceptance and sense of community whereas women used words representing social and affective processes.[14] When comparing by race/ethnicity, this work showed that minority applicants wrote with more clout, a measure of confidence compared to white applicants.[15]

Given conscious efforts to improve diversity and inclusion within urology in conjunction with the increased importance of personal statements due to the impact of COVID on visiting rotations and in-person interviews, we sought to assess whether personal statement linguistics have changed in response to ongoing initiatives. The personal statement serves as a core component of the urology application. It represents a one-page essay that gives the applicant a chance to introduce themselves and their career interests to a reader who will ultimately decide on whether to grant an interview offer. We hypothesized that linguistics differences by gender and race/ethnicity have narrowed from 2016-2017 to 2022-2023. Differences discovered in the subtelties of personal statement linguistics may offer early objective data regarding the success of diversity and inclusion efforts to address disparities in the urologic workforce.

Materials and methods

Study Cohort and Procedure

After receiving IRB approval, applications to the Department of Urology residency program at the University of North Carolina at Chapel Hill during the 2016-2017 and 2022-2023 application cycles were extracted from the Electronic Residency Application Service (ERAS) platform and de-identified. Demographic data of applicants were manually extracted from the residency applications, including age, race/ethnicity, and gender. The study team also ascertained the number of gap years between medical school and residency, United States Medical Licensing Exam (USMLE) Step 1 score, number of research projects, and medical school. Finally, the study team extracted the personal statement from each application. Current application guidelines limit personal statements to 3500 characters.

Primary Exposures

Self-identified gender and race/ethnicity in the Electronic Residency Application Service application served as the primary exposures. For the analysis, we initially categorized gender as male, female, non-binary, and non-reported. Due to the very small number of applicants selecting non-binary or non-reported, we limited our analysis to those identifying as female or male. We categorized race/ethnicity into three categories: non-Hispanic White (NHW), Asian, and URMs. We designated Asians separately as they are not considered to be underrepresented in urology though still may be subject to conscious and unconscious bias.[16] The URM group included those identifying as Black, Latinx/Hispanic or of Spanish origin, Native American, Native Alaskan, or Pacific Islander. To be consistent with our prior analysis, we also included "Other" or non-reported race within the URM group.[15] As a sensitivity analysis, we also tested an alternative race/ethnicity categorization that limited URMs to Black, Latinx/Hispanic or of Spanish origin, Native American, Native Alaskan, or Pacific Islander.

Covariates

Age, USMLE Step 1 score, number of gap years between medical school and residency, and number of research projects were treated as continuous variables. Using data from the U.S. News & World Report Best Medical School Research rankings for 2017 and 2022,[17] we created a binary measure for medical school rank in the top 25 vs. all others. Finally, we created a binary variable for application cycle (2022–2023 vs. 2016–2017).

Primary Outcomes

The linguistic qualities of applicants' personal statements served as the primary outcomes, which were measured using the 2022 version of the Linguistic Inquiry and Word Count (LIWC), an internally and externally validated text analysis program (Pennebaker Conglomerates, Inc, Austin TX).[18] Compared to the 2015 version used previously,[14,15] the most current LIWC program utilizes an expanded word dictionary and includes new word categories related to linguistics as well as themes. Like the previous version, the LIWC reports the word count, 4 summary language variables (analytical thinking, clout, authenticity, and emotional tone), as well as multiple word categories and subdomains. Each summary language variable is a research-based composite score created using a proprietary algorithm. Their value, assigned on a 0-100 scale, quantifies text characteristics. The analytic thinking score describes how rational and formal text is. Clout refers to writing that is authoritative, confident and exhibits leadership. Authenticity refers to writing that is personal and honest. A higher emotional tone score describes positive emotions while lower scores describe more negative writing. Word categories and subdomains determine what percentage of the analyzed text contains words referencing different language categories,

Table 1
LICW word categories and subdomain

Category	Description or Most Frequent Example
Word Count	Total word count
Analytic	Metric of logical, formal thinking
Clout	Language of leadership, status
Authenticity	Perceived honesty, genuineness
Tone	Degree of positive (negative) tone
Linguistic	Subdomain representing variables of words
Drives	We, our, work, us
Cognition	Way people think or refer to thinking (is, was, but, are)
Differentiation	But, not, if, or
Affect	Good, well, new, love
Tone Negative	Bad, wrong, too much, hate
Emotion	Good, love, happy, hope
Positive Emotion	Good, love, happy, hope
Negative Emotion	Bad, hate, hurt, tired
Social Processes	Seeks to reflect broad sets of social behaviors (you, we, he, she)
Social Behavior	Signal helping or caring about others (said, love, say, care)
Moralization	Wrong, honor, deserve, judge
Social Referents	you, we, he, she
Culture	Overarching dimension of politics, ethnicity, technology
Politics	Words commonly used in political or legal discourse (United states, govern, congress, senate)
Ethnicity	Identify national, regional, ethnic, or racial identities (American, French, Chinese, Indian)
Technology	Refers to scientific or technologic devices (car, phone, computer, email)
Lifestyle	work, home, school, working
Leisure	Game, fun, play, party
Home	Home, house, room, bed
Work	Work, school, working, class
Religion	God, hell, Christmas, church
Physical	Medic, food, patients, eye
Death	Death, dead, die, kill
Motives – Reward	Underlying states that guide, drive, pull behavior (opportunity, win, gain, benefit)
Motives – Allure	Words used in ads or persuasive communication (have, like, out, know)
Perceptions	Refers to sensory or perceptual dimensions related to 5 senses (in, out, up, there)

psychological constructs, or themes (**Table 1**). Categories either significantly updated or newly introduced for the 2022 version include cognition (ways people think), affect, social behavior, culture (eg, politics, ethnicity, technology), and motives.

Statistical Analysis

First, we compared applicant characteristics by gender and race/ethnicity using parametric and non-parametric testing as appropriate. For each linguistic quality, we then fit multivariable regression models with race/ethnicity, gender, and application cycle to estimate the baseline main effects. Next, we conducted a difference-in-differences analysis to assess differential change in linguistic qualities of personal statements by gender and race/ethnicity between application cycles. Difference-in-differences is a quasi-experimental study design that controls for secular trends and has been increasingly used to assess the impact of policy in surgical health services research.[19] Statistically, it assesses for a differential change by adding and evaluating an interaction term between the pre-post periods (ie, application cycle) and exposures of interest (ie, gender, race/ethnicity) to the baseline model, which were evaluated here in two separate models. Finally, to assess the robustness of our findings, we performed two sensitivity analyses (ie, distinguishing between traditional URMs and "Other"/non-reported, adjusting for USMLE Step 1 score and top 25 medical school).

Statistical analyses were performed using R Statistical Software (v4.1.1; R Core Team 2021) with significance set at the 0.05 level.

RESULTS

The analysis included 342 applications from the 2016-2017 cycle and 425 applications from 2022 to 2023 cycle. When combined, a total of 257 applicants were female making up 33.5% of applicants while 184 were classified as URMs, representing 24.0% of all applicants. Applicant characteristics by gender and race/ethnicity are reported in **Tables 2** and **3**, respectively. Of note, a greater proportion of female (23.3%) and URM (23.9%) applicants attended a medical school ranked in the top 25 compared to male (16.8%) and NHW (13.5%) applicants. Additionally, females and URMs scored slightly lower on the USMLE Step 1 exam compared to males and NHWs, respectively.

When evaluating the summary variables of word count, analytic thinking, clout, authenticity, and emotional tone across the two cycles, a few differences emerged by gender, race/ethnicity, and year. In the baseline main effects model without interactions (**Table 4**), female applicants wrote with more clout (+1.87, p = 0.03) compared to their male counterparts. For URMs, their personal statements had higher word counts (+24.42, p = 0.03) but scored with less authenticity (−2.96, p = 0.03) compared to NHWs. Adjusting for gender and race/ethnicity, emotional tone (−2.61, p = 0.02) also decreased between application cycles.

When evaluating the word categories and subdomains, there were several differences with respect to gender and race/ethnicity (see **Table 4**). Compared to male applicants, female applicants wrote with increased emotion (+0.13 p = 0.01), specifically increased negative emotion (+0.07 p = 0.01). Female applicants also made more references to social processes (+0.80 p = 0.00) and social behavior (+0.33 p = 0.00). Lastly, female applicants' personal statements had decreased verbiage relating to technology (−0.10 p = 0.00) or home (−0.07 p = 0.01). Compared to NHW applicants, URM applicants had more social

Table 2
Applicant characteristics overall and by gender

Characteristic	Overall	Male (N = 507)	Female (N = 257)	P-value
Age (years)	27.0 (SD 2.9)	27.5 (SD 2.9)	27.3 (SD 2.8)	0.58
Race				
Non-Hispanic White	422 (55.2%)	286 (56.4%)	136 (52.9%)	0.14
Asian	160 (20.9%)	111 (21.9%)	49 (19.1%)	
URM	182 (23.8%)	110 (21.7%)	72 (28.0%)	
Top 25 Medical School	145 (19.0%)	85 (16.8%)	60 (23.3%)	0.04
Gap Years	1.5 (SD 1.9)	1.4 (SD 1.9)	1.7 (SD 1.9)	0.03
Research Projects	7.7 (SD 7.8)	7.8 (SD 8.4)	7.5 (SD 6.6)	0.47
USMLE Step 1 Score	241.9 (SD 14.2)	243.1 (SD 14.3)	239.4 (SD 13.5)	<0.01

Abbreviation: URM, underrepresented minorities in medicine including other or non-reported

Table 3
Applicant characteristics by race/ethnicity

Characteristic	NHW (N = 423)	Asian (N = 160)	URM (N = 184)	P-value
Age (years)	27.3 (SD 2.3)	27.0 (SD 3.1)	28.0 (SD 3.7)	<0.01
Top 25 Medical School	57 (13.5%)	44 (27.5%)	44 (23.9%)	<0.01
Gap Years	1.6 (SD 1.9)	1.2 (SD 1.7)	1.7 (SD 2.0)	0.05
Research Projects	6.9 (SD 6.8)	9.3 (SD 8.0)	8.2 (SD 9.5)	<0.01
USMLE Step 1 Score	243.3 (SD 12.6)	243.8 (SD 13.0)	236.7 (SD 17.4)	<0.01

Abbreviations: NHW, non-Hispanic White; URM, underrepresented minorities in medicine including other or non-reported.

processes seen in their writing (+0.58 p = 0.00) as well as more moralization (+0.04, p = 0.02). Notably, URMs showed a statistically significant increase in cultural (+0.33 p = 0.00), political (+0.17 p = 0.00), and ethnicity (+0.14, p = 0.00) references in their personal statements. Lastly, URM personal statements saw less use of words reflecting leisure (−0.11, p = 0.01) and motives/allure (−0.28, p = 0.01).

We observed several differences in linguistic qualities between application cycles. Compared to 2016-2017, personal statements in 2022-2023 had increased negative tone (+0.18, p = 0.00) and negative emotion (+0.08, p = 0.00). Personal statements also made more social process references in the 2022-2023 cycle (+0.58, p = 0.00), particularly social behavior (+0.39, p = 0.00), moralization (+0.03, p = 0.04), and social referents (+0.45, p = 0.00). Applicants in 2022-2023 also made less reference to their lifestyle (−0.64, p = 0.00), particularly work (−0.67, p = 0.00), though with slightly more mention of ethnicity (+0.05, p = 0.00).

In the difference-in-difference analysis, very few linguistic qualities changed differently between cycles by gender or race/ethnicity (see **Table 4**). For both female and URM applicants, we observed no differences in trends for analytic thinking, clout, authenticity, or emotional tone compared to male and NHW applicants, respectively. Female applicants had a decrease in linguistic score (−1.39, p = 0.02) and use of differentiation (−0.28, p = 0.02) and motives/allure (−0.36, p < 0.05) words relative to male applicants. Compared to NHW personal statements, URM personal statements increased in moralization (+0.10, p = 0.00) and references to ethnicity (+0.13, p = 0.00) and a decreased in references to technology (−0.22, p = 0.00). In the two sensitivity analyses, the differences noted for clout among females, word count and authenticity among URMs, and emotional tone in the 2022-2023 cycle did not reach statistical significance but remained similar in effect size and directionality. The remaining findings did not differ substantively.

DISCUSSION

Diversity and inclusion in the urologic force remains an ongoing challenge and priority with multiple local and national initiatives underway. Because these efforts are directed mostly toward trainees, studying the linguistic qualities of personal statements may offer an early snapshot into the impact of these programs. Examining personal statements from 2016-2017 and 2022-2023, we found that female applicants wrote with more clout and emotion compared to male applicants while URM applicants made more cultural references yet scored lower on authenticity compared to NWH applicants. However, we observed very few changes in linguistic qualities by gender or race/ethnicity over time, suggesting that ongoing initiatives may not have had a sizable impact on the application process, at least in this regard.

Multiple prior studies have performed linguistic analyses of components of graduate medical education applications. As noted above, in our prior analysis, males used words that indicated acceptance and sense of community whereas women used words representing social and affective processes.[14] This is similar to our current study showing that female applicants mention more social processes in their writing use more words representing negative emotions such as bad, hurt, wrong. A 2019 study investigated personal statements from pediatric residency interviewees, finding that males used agentic (self-oriented) language of reward more frequently than their female counterparts.[20] A similar study in 2017 evaluated the personal statements for general surgery applicants, noting that women tended to discuss surgery as a team endeavor while men more commonly focused on their personal surgical experiences.[21] A fourth paper, published in 2018, performed language comparisons on the letters

Table 4
Changes in linguistic qualities by exposure

Linguistic Quality[a]	Main Effects			Interactions	
	Δfemale	ΔURM	Δyear	Δfemale_year	ΔURM_year
Word Count	+16.19 (0.09)	+24.42 (0.03)	+5.31 (0.56)	−28.87 (0.13)	−7.76 (0.73)
Analytical	−0.96 (0.25)	+1.15 (0.24)	−0.98 (0.22)	+2.38 (0.16)	+1.13 (0.57)
Clout	+1.87 (0.03)	+1.17 (0.24)	+1.29 (0.12)	+3.26 (0.06)	−0.86 (0.67)
Authenticity	−1.18 (0.33)	−2.96 (0.03)	+1.56 (0.18)	−3.07 (0.21)	−3.79 (0.18)
Tone	−0.33 (0.78)	−0.68 (0.62)	−2.61 (0.02)	+1.75 (0.47)	−1.16 (0.68)
Linguistic	−0.28 (0.34)	−0.62 (0.06)	−0.18 (0.53)	−1.39 (0.02)	−0.65 (0.34)
Drives	+0.12 (0.37)	+0.15 (0.33)	+0.14 (0.28)	+0.04 (0.88)	+0.40 (0.19)
Cognition	−0.08 (0.61)	−0.11 (0.54)	+0.05 (0.71)	−0.23 (0.46)	−0.25 (0.48)
Differentiation	+0.03 (0.59)	+0.01 (0.91)	+0.20 (0.00)	−0.28 (0.02)	−0.04 (0.77)
Affect	+0.12 (0.20)	+0.01 (0.91)	+0.10 (0.25)	−0.04 (0.83)	+0.36 (0.09)
Tone Negative	+0.07 (0.08)	+0.04 (0.47)	+0.18 (0.00)	−0.12 (0.15)	+0.19 (0.06)
Emotion	+0.13 (0.01)	−0.03 (0.54)	−0.03 (0.50)	−0.05 (0.61)	+0.00 (0.99)
Positive Emotion	+0.05 (0.13)	−0.06 (0.13)	−0.09 (0.01)	+0.02 (0.79)	−0.13 (0.12)
Negative Emotion	+0.07 (0.01)	+0.03 (0.39)	+0.08 (0.00)	−0.08 (0.14)	+0.11 (0.08)
Social Processes	+0.80 (0.00)	+0.58 (0.00)	+0.92 (0.00)	+0.27 (0.45)	+0.20 (0.63)
Social Behavior	+0.33 (0.00)	+0.21 (0.03)	+0.39 (0.00)	+0.08 (0.65)	+0.12 (0.55)
Moralization	+0.01 (0.71)	+0.04 (0.02)	+0.03 (0.04)	+0.05 (0.13)	+0.10 (0.00)
Social Referents	+0.47 (0.00)	+0.25 (0.09)	+0.45 (0.00)	+0.25 (0.33)	+0.02 (0.96)
Culture	−0.05 (0.21)	+0.33 (0.00)	+0.04 (0.35)	+0.03 (0.72)	−0.14 (0.16)
Politics	+0.03 (0.17)	+0.17 (0.00)	+0.01 (0.77)	+0.05 (0.26)	−0.03 (0.59)
Ethnicity	+0.02 (0.28)	+0.14 (0.00)	+0.05 (0.00)	+0.04 (0.23)	+0.13 (0.00)
Technology	−0.10 (0.00)	+0.04 (0.26)	−0.01 (0.78)	−0.04 (0.53)	−0.22 (0.00)
Lifestyle	−0.28 (0.06)	−0.19 (0.28)	−0.64 (0.00)	+0.20 (0.52)	+0.03 (0.94)
Leisure	−0.07 (0.09)	−0.11 (0.01)	−0.02 (0.66)	+0.00 (1.00)	+0.11 (0.25)
Home	−0.07 (0.01)	−0.02 (0.52)	−0.02 (0.35)	−0.03 (0.53)	−0.06 (0.38)
Work	−0.16 (0.26)	−0.07 (0.65)	−0.63 (0.00)	+0.22 (0.45)	−0.20 (0.56)
Religion	+0.01 (0.49)	+0.00 (0.91)	+0.02 (0.04)	−0.00 (0.99)	−0.01 (0.51)
Physical	+0.14 (0.22)	+0.12 (0.38)	−0.01 (0.95)	+0.38 (0.11)	+0.37 (0.18)
Death	+0.01 (0.18)	+0.02 (0.02)	−0.01 (0.20)	−0.01 (0.62)	−0.00 (0.84)
Motives – Reward	−0.05 (0.11)	−0.01 (0.84)	−0.05 (0.06)	+0.09 (0.13)	+0.07 (0.31)
Motives – Allure	+0.12 (0.19)	−0.28 (0.01)	−0.04 (0.65)	−0.36 (0.05)	+0.10 (0.62)
Perceptions	−0.08 (0.46)	−0.22 (0.10)	+0.46 (0.00)	−0.24 (0.29)	−0.18 (0.49)

Abbreviations: URM, underrepresented minorities in medicine including other or non-reported.

[a] Δfemale, ΔURM, Δyear beta estimates (p-value) from base model. Δfemale_year beta estimate (p-value) from main effects model + gender by year interaction term. ΔURM_year beta estimate (p-value) from main effects model + race by year interaction term.

of recommendation for general surgery applicants and reported that female writers wrote longer letters than male writers and "standout" terms were more likely to be used to describe female applicants.[22] In some respects, these studies suggest that female applicants write their personal statements in manners that conform to preexisting gender norms, perhaps perpetuating stereotypes.

While our findings indicate that personal statements from female applicants have remained relatively unchanged from our previous analysis, we observe one notable exception. In this iteration, personal statements from female applicants had higher clout scores. Though not statistically significant, the difference appears to be driven by the most current cycle. This difference may reflect a changed perception of the "outsider" status of female applicants in urology and greater confidence in their candidacy. From 2007 to 2019, the number of practicing female urologists increased 10.4%.[23] Female residents now account for 25% of urology residents and 37% of our most recent application cohort.[24] In 2022, 72% of female applicants matched compared with only 63% of male applicants.[25] Collectively, these trends may reflect increased female mentorship and the impact of programming centered around increasing gender diversity in the urologic workforce.

To the best of our knowledge, no prior study besides ours has analyzed the impact of race/ethnicity on the linguistics of personal statements. However, there has been some linguistic evaluation of letters of recommendation for applicants to various specialties within medicine. A 2021 study in obstetrics and gynecology evaluated whether linguistic differences existed in letters of recommendation for residency applications based on race, noting that White and Asian applicants more often received comments on surgical skills, leadership, and work ethic compared to URM applicants.[26] An analysis of 4 years of applicant data from 2015 to 2019 within radiation oncology residencies found that letters of recommendation for URM applicants were significantly less likely to include standout descriptors such as "superb" and "remarkable."[27] When expressing themselves though, URMs less often used leisure words and made more references to social processes including moralization that signal high virtue, which could be desirable qualities for surgery and surgical specialties.

Of note, URMs used more words about culture, politics, and ethnicity compared to NHWs with increasing use of ethnicity words over time. Between application cycles, many pivotal and national news events occurred, which brought racial injustices in American to the forefront. Black Lives Matters and White Coat for Black Lives shared many demonstrations of solidarity and set many health care institutions on a path toward more inclusive cultures.[28,29] During this movement, URMs may have felt more empowered to express their culture and ethnicity in their personal statements. It may also explain the increased political language as well. However, despite more URM dedicated programs and broader initiatives to increase diversity in urology, only 51% of URM applicants matched in the 2022 cycle compared to 65% of White applicants and 69% of Asian applicant.[25] Paradoxically, URM personal statements received lower authenticity scores despite more mentions of culture, politics, and ethnicity. As one possible explanation, increased self-expression by URMs in personal statements

may yield mixed results depending on the perspectives of the reader, highlighting the need to address biases more broadly while also promoting URM-specific programming to increase diversity and inclusion in the urologic workforce.

The relative lack of change in personal statement linguistics over time despite ongoing initiatives directed toward female and URM applicants could reflect the overriding disruptions to the application process caused by COVID-19. For 2022-2023 applicants, their medical school education was conducted largely in the shadow of COVID, affecting their didactic and experiential instruction. These applicants had fewer total research projects compared to those in 2017, which may be due to reduced networking opportunities with members of urology departments, as classes and interest group events were cancelled or moved online. There is extremely limited data on how COVID-19 impacted residency applications with regards to personal statements. In one 2022 study of 31 orthopedic surgery residency programs, 8 "put more weight" on personal statements tailored to their specific program while 2 gave more consideration to the personal statement overall.[30] At the same time, personal statements likely have gained even greater importance from the perspective of the applicants. With reduced opportunities for in-person meetings and away rotations, the written portion of the application became one of the few mechanisms by which applicants can affect the application process. Accordingly, we see several linguistic differences between cycles relating to overall tone, emotion, social processes, and lifestyle.

The results of this study must be viewed in the context of several limitations. First, it is possible that the LIWC program may misinterpret the tone and intent of personal statements to some degree, particularly as it relates to medical language. LIWC may also be subject to inherent biases as seen with other computer algorithms and programs.[31] Second, we used a broader definition of URM that included "other" and missing race/ethnicity to be consistent with our prior analysis.[15] Notably, our findings did not differ substantively when using a stricter definition of URM. Third, while we can identify differences, establishing a causal relationship with observational data remains elusive. As noted in **Tables 2** and **3**, some differences exist in applicant characteristics by gender and race/ethnicity. However, our findings did not differ substantively when adjusting for USMLE Step 1 score and top 25 medical school. Furthermore, the inclusion of a difference-in-differences analysis may offer some quasi-experimental qualities though residual confounding from concurrent events likely remains, particularly from COVID-19. Even in the absence of competing events, our design assesses the broader environment and not the effectiveness of individual programs. Fourth, this study does not include match data, as used in our previous study. Therefore, the impact of these minor linguistic differences on applicant perception and ultimately match results remain speculative. Fifth, our data may not be generalizable to all urology residency applicants since this is a study from a single institution. However, we captured 425 of 556 (76.4%) of total applications for the 2022-2023 cycle, indicating relative high sample of the total pool.[25] Lastly, letters of recommendation were not examined in this study, and they may represent an even stronger source of gender- and race-based differences as demonstrated by prior studies from different medical specialties such as gynecology and surgery.[22,26,27]

These limitations notwithstanding, these linguistic differences offer a small window into the potential impact of ongoing diversity and inclusion initiatives in urology. For female applicants, these findings in conjunction with higher match rates may serve as a sign of early success. Female applicants continue to write with more emotion and social process references but now express more clout, which may be driven by the increased visibility of women in urology and concerted efforts to provide mentorship and ensure inclusion. However, similar trends were not observed for URMs. Whereas URMs more often used words relating to culture, ethnicity, and politics, their personal statements generated lower authenticity scores, and they experienced a lower match rate in the 2022-2023 cycle than NHWs. These findings highlight the need for continued efforts to engage, mentor, coach, and sponsor URM applicants, so they represent themselves strongly in their applications and overcome biases that may persist in the application process itself. Studies have shown the beneficial impact of a diverse workforce on patient satisfaction, with racial and gender concordance between patients and physicians being linked to higher patient experience scores.[32] Our study indicates that work remains, especially to increase the number of URMs entering urology.

SUMMARY

Modest linguistic differences in personal statements exist for female and URM applicants to urology compared to their male and NHW counterparts, respectively. Whereas female applicants now write with more clout and have increased presence in the urologic workforce, the linguistic differences for URMs may be vulnerable to ongoing biases that negatively impact entrance into urology. These findings suggest that more needs to be done to ensure URM medical students have avenues for gaining exposure to urology and opportunities for sponsorship and mentorship, so all applicants feel welcomed and appreciated in the field.

REFERENCES

1. *Census results - American Urological Association.* (2022) [Report]. American Urological Association (AUA). Available at: https://www.auanet.org/research-and-data/aua-census/census-results.
2. U.S. Census Bureau QuickFacts: *United States.* (2022). Census Bureau QuickFacts. Available at: https://www.census.gov/quickfacts/fact/table/US/PST045222. Accessed July 1, 2022.
3. Urologists in Training: *Residents and Fellows In the United States.* (2021). [Report]. American Urological Association (AUA).
4. Owens-Walton J, Cooley KAL, Herbert AS, et al. Solutions: bridging the diversity gap in urology trainees. Urology 2022;162:121–7.
5. Simons ECG, Arevalo A, Washington SL, et al. Trends in the racial and ethnic diversity in the US urology workforce. Urology 2022;162:9–19.
6. Barquin D, Tella D, Tuong M, et al. Factors influencing underrepresented in medicine urologist recruitment to academic institutions. Urol Pract 2023;10(2):187–92.
7. AUA announces Diversity and Inclusion Task Force. American Urological Association MediaRoom. December 22, 2020. Available at: https://auanet.mediaroom.com/2020-12-22-AUA-Announces-Diversity-and-Inclusion-Task-Force. Accessed March 3 2023.
8. Adam Hittelman. Taskforce Update: Attracting Women and Underrepresented Minorities (URMS) to Urology. Presented at SAU Program Directors, Coordinators & Academicians Meeting; February 1, 2019.
9. Cannon S, Seideman CA, Thavaseelan S, et al. Urologists for equity: a collective approach toward diversity, equity, and inclusion in urology. Urology 2022; 162:33–7.
10. "Explore Urim Opportunities for Visiting Students." Students & Residents, Available at: students-residents.aamc.org/students/explore-urim-opportunities-visiting-students. Accessed 14 May 2023.
11. "Sub-Internship Information." UCSF Department of Urology, Available at: urology.ucsf.edu/education/residency/sub-internship-information. Accessed 14 May 2023.
12. Diversity Visiting Student Sub-Internship Program." Department of Urology, Available at: urology.uw.

edu/education/medical-students/diversity-sub-internship. Accessed 14 May 2023.

13. Underrepresented Minority Medical Students." Pennmedicine.Org, Available at: www.pennmedicine.org/departments-and-centers/department-of-surgery/education-and-training/medical-students/urim-clerkship. Accessed 14 May 2023.

14. Demzik A, Filippou P, Chew C, et al. Gender-based differences in urology residency applicant personal statements. Urology 2021;150:2–8.

15. Demzik A, Filippou P, Chew C, et al. Linguistic differences in personal statements of urology residency applicants by self-reported race and ethnicity. Urology 2022;162:137–43.

16. Clay WA, Jackson DH, Harris KA. Does the AAMC's definition of "underrepresented in medicine" promote justice and inclusivity? AMA J Ethics 2021; 23(12):E960–4.

17. 2022 Best Medical Schools: Research. US News and World Report. Available at: https://www.usnews.com/best-graduate-schools/top-medical-schools/research-rankings. Accessed March 3, 2023.

18. Boyd RL, Ashokkumar A, Seraj S, et al. The development and psychometric properties of LIWC-22. Austin, TX: University of Texas at Austin; 2022. Available at: https://www.liwc.app.

19. Dimick JB, Ryan AM. Methods for evaluating changes in health care policy: the difference-in-differences approach. JAMA 2014;312(22):2401–2.

20. Babal JC, Gower AD, Frohna JG, et al. Linguistic analysis of pediatric residency personal statements: gender differences. BMC Med Educ 2019;19(1): 392.

21. Ostapenko L, Schonhardt-Bailey C, Sublette JW, et al. Textual analysis of general surgery residency personal statements: topics and gender differences. J Surg Educ 2018;75(3):573–81.

22. French JC, Zolln SJ, Lampert E, et al. Gender and letters of recommendation: a linguistic comparison of the impact of gender on general surgery residency applicants. J Surg Educ 2019;76(4):899–905.

23. Findlay BL, Bearrick EN, Granberg CF, et al. Path to parity: trends in female representation among physicians, trainees, and applicants in urology and surgical specialties. Urology 2023;172:228–33.

24. Nam CS, Daignault-Newton S, Herrel LA, et al. The future is female: urology workforce projection from 2020 to 2060. Urology 2021;150:30–4.

25. Match Statistics: 2022 Urology Residency Match. (2022). [Report]. American Urological Association (AUA).

26. Brown O, Mou T, Lim SI, et al. Do gender and racial differences exist in letters of recommendation for obstetrics and gynecology residency applicants? Am J Obstet Gynecol 2021;225(5):554.e1–11.

27. Chapman BV, Rooney MK, Ludmir EB, et al. Linguistic biases in letters of recommendation for radiation oncology residency applicants from 2015 to 2019. J Cancer Educ 2022;37(4):965–72.

28. Nguyen BM, Guh J, Freeman B. Black lives matter: moving from passion to action in academic medical institutions. J Natl Med Assoc 2022;114(2):193–8.

29. Sullivan C, Quaintance J, Myers T, et al. A framework to support medical students' professional development during large-scale societal events. Acad Psychiatry 2023;1–6. https://doi.org/10.1007/s40596-023-01795-5.

30. Khalafallah YM, Markowitz M, Levine WN, et al. Orthopaedic surgery residency application, and selection criteria adaptations, in times of COVID-19: a survey study. JB JS Open Access 2022;7(2). e21. 00145.

31. Garcia M. Racist in the machine: the disturbing implications of algorithmic bias. World Pol J 2016; 33(4):111–7. Available at: https://www.jstor.org/stable/26781452.

32. Burton É, Flores B, Jerome B, et al. Assessment of bias in patient safety reporting systems categorized by physician gender, race and ethnicity, and faculty rank: a qualitative study. JAMA Netw Open 2022; 5(5):e2213234.

Clinical Care and Education around Diverse Patient Populations

The Role of Diversity, Equity, and Inclusion Principles in Enhancing the Quality of Urologic Resident Education and Advancing Gender Diverse Care

Christi Butler, MD

KEYWORDS

- Trauma informed care • Transgender and gender diverse • Diversity, equity, and inclusion
- Implicit bias

KEY POINTS

- Health disparities are prevalent among the trans and gender diverse community.
- Disparities are rooted in a system that is designed to discriminate and bias against trans and gender diverse individuals.
- Diversity, equity, and inclusion (DEI) programs may help increase and change behavior towards how we treat trans and gender diverse individuals.

INTRODUCTION

Urologists have a unique role in their care as genitourinary specialists as they will undoubtedly encounter transgender and gender diverse (TGD) patients with urinary and sexual problems. As urologists, it is important that we should be aware of the issues that TGD, and other minority groups alike, face, and how we can best address it through incorporation of education among ourselves and trainees. For too long the medical field has effectively neglected those from minority and diverse backgrounds. This has been more than evident in how research has been conducted and the presence of existing health disparities within urology.[1,2] In turn, this has had an impact on *who* we treat and *how* we treat as practitioners. Interestingly, even the little research that has been done on disparities in urology largely focuses on race and cis women and rarely the lesbian, gay, bisexual, trans, queer plus (LGBTQ+) population. Proposed mechanisms to combat these disparities include increased access for underserved populations, increased representation of underrepresented health care providers and education.[3] With regard to education, there is a push to include and improve a diversity, equity, and inclusion focused curriculum. This is particularly important when considering how urology, as a field, may improve from not only a health outcome perspective, but as a means of better serving patients as a whole. This article will discuss the importance of diversity, equity, and inclusion (DEI) education programs, with a particular focus on the needs of the TGD community.

THE PROBLEM

It is estimated that TGD individuals make up roughly 0.6% of the US population, with 25 million

Note: race/ethnicity–denotes that both race and ethnicity were combined in this analysis, but that race and ethnicity are distinctly different and not synonymous.
University of California San Francisco, 400 Parnassus Avenue, 6th Floor, San Francisco, CA 94143, USA
E-mail address: Christi.Butler@ucsf.edu

individuals identifying worldwide.[4] Unfortunately, the TGD community has faced pervasive discrimination, rejection, and even violence in society as a whole, as well as, within the field of medicine.[5–7] When it comes to the TGD community and more broadly those from the gender and sexual minority (GSM) community, there has been a longstanding existence of disparities. Although there are a multitude of contributing barriers in place, many of these disparities are rooted in trans and queerphobia. Such prejudices and discrimination have led TGD patients to internal stigmas, mistrust, and expectations of negative experiences, which, unfortunately, result in poorer health outcomes[8,9] Specifically, 33% of TGD patients reported a negative experience in the medical field.[5] In a qualitative study, individuals have reported experiences of misgendering, looks of confusion, irrelevant invasive questioning, improper documentation, and the burden of educating providers.[10] Further, a 2012 study conducted by Harvard Kennedy School found that trans-identifying patients experienced medical care refusal at a rate of 14% to 20%.[11] This, in conjunction with a history of denial for insurance coverage, a lack of providers equipped to treat TGD patients, and a culturally incompetent health system, has resulted in patients avoiding medical care.[12]

Additionally, the TGD have been absent from most patient-centered research resulting in a lack of knowledge and patient-reported outcomes in this population. In a review performed by Sineath and colleagues,[8] they found that only 45 urology-related articles included members from sexual gender minority (SGM) group. Within that group, they identified 17 different scales used for patient-reported outcomes, of which only 3 had been validated. They also found that there was a paucity of engagement of the SGM community and underrepresentation in many urologic disease research areas. Lack of inclusion in research only further isolates them as a patient population and limits how to best incorporate or interpret new, health-improving information when treating these patients specifically.

BARRIERS

When considering how to address these health care inequities, one must first understand the barriers that are in place for the TGD community. Largely, these barriers can be broken into the following categories: clinical environment including health care system design and health care team interactions, patient-specific restrictions, and provider mindset. From a clinical perspective, a multitude of studies across specialties have identified a

lack of inclusivity in documentation and health care forms.[10,13,14] For example, many health records and documentation default to using pronouns or language associated with one's assigned sex at birth and are often unrelated to TGD specific health needs. Staff may incorrectly provide a "standard health form" that more relates to a cis-gender person with a focus on specific anatomy that the patient finds distressing or uncomfortable for them. This can lead to a propagation of inappropriate assumptions and poor interactions causing a patient to feel unwelcome and no longer desire to seek care at that clinic. This is especially relevant in a urologic setting where the focus is on genitourinary health and an accurate account of one's anatomy is crucial to caring for addressing patient's issue.

Regarding patient-specific restrictions, it is no secret that today's political environment has become quite divisive with many political activists targeting health care for sexual minority and TGD members. In 2023 alone there have been over 500 anti-trans bills proposed, with at least 140 proposed bills specific to health care.[15,16] The effect of such legislature is the looming threat of criminalization, license revocation, or high fines for "violation," which include offering and/or managing patients seeking gender affirming care. Although the majority of these bans have targeted trans youth, the rise in bills have instilled a fear among all patients and providers alike. The consequences are life threatening and have already started to occur in some cases: for example, insurance companies may withdraw care coverage for TGD individuals, providers offering care may become more scarce, and patients may be forced to travel long distances to find providers in safe haven locations, seek unsanctioned alternatives, or opt to avoid seeking care altogether.

There may also be a high level of discomfort with caring for TGD individuals among providers that serve as an additional barrier. Sineath and colleagues[8] suggested that transphobia may be a barrier to educating providers on trans-related care as further supported by a recent survey by Stroumsa and colleagues[17] that found that knowledge of trans health care had a negative correlation with transphobia. Interestingly, both Stroumsa and colleagues[17] and Kent and colleagues[18] found no correlation between provider comfort with formal trans education, but more so with prior experience and willingness to care for trans folks. This would suggest that one's attitude towards the TGD community serve as an even bigger barrier to receiving equal and just care. One contributing factor to discriminatory behavior is through one's own personal bias, which can be either explicit (deliberate) or implicit (unconscious). Unconscious or implicit bias is defined as associations or attitudes that can impact our judgment, behavior, and actions, which can cause a dissociation from what a person explicitly claims to believe.[19] According to Marcelin and colleagues,[20] underrepresented minorities are the most vulnerable to unconscious bias that are derived from cultural stereotypes and perpetuate health disparities that can negatively impact patient–clinician interactions. That being said, the history and cultural nuances of the TGD community is not something that is widely taught in today's medical curriculum. Much like what has been seen in other marginalized communities, a lack of understanding of the history of the TGD can be a poor set up for the patient–provider relationship, which is so critical to perceived experience and adherence to medical advice.[21–23] There is an opportunity here for improvement.

CURRENT TRANSGENDER AND GENDER DIVERSE EDUCATION AMONG TRAINEES

The inclusion of transgender health has not traditionally been a part of medical training and continues to remain notably lacking in medical school curricula.[24] Consequently, there is a gap in the knowledge and understanding of the history of TGD individuals in health care among current and rising health care providers. As previously mentioned, this lends itself towards discriminatory behavior that can further isolate the TGD population and negatively impact their overall health. It has been well supported that education and understanding is imperative especially at the student and trainee level. A qualitative study found that TGD-identifying individuals were more likely to trust and have confidence in their health care provider who had knowledge and competency in TGD health and who provided a dedicated LGBTQ + positive space.[10]

Urology, unlike many other surgical specialties, is unique in that TGD patients may seek our care not only for general urologic problems but also to seek specific gender affirming surgical services. However, this is not widely taught or available in most training programs. Research has shown that only one-quarter of plastic surgery residencies and less than half of obstetric and gynecological residencies have had exposure or any formal training or didactics in trans-related care.[25,26] In a survey that specifically looked at urological programs, 42% of responding programs reported having no transgender dedicated didactics and 30% of programs provided no clinical exposure.[27] Whether or not program directors chose to incorporate

trans-related didactics was associated with their attitude towards the value of trans care. Again, this speaks to the importance of exposure, behavior adjustment, and proper education. By ignoring these fundamental and necessary principles in our trainee educational experience, we are doing a disservice to our TGD patients.

IMPORTANCE OF DIVERSITY EQUITY AND INCLUSION

Breaking down the barriers to care is not easy and requires participation and investment at all levels. As urologists, we can have an impact through dedicated efforts to combat any cultural knowledge gaps and address any inequities or discriminatory behavior head on. One such effort is through implementation of DEI programs. According to the World Health Organization, the purpose of DEI programs is to "provide strategic leadership on the [social determinants of health and equity by] developing evidence, norms and standards."[28] Education and recruitment efforts centered in DEI allows us to specifically learn about and potentially address underlying issues that have led to health disparities in the first place. Improvements in diversity have been shown to improve health outcomes in Black and LatinX/Hispanic patient populations by improving access to care, communication, trust, understanding of cultural differences and potential barriers, patient satisfaction, and inclusivity.[29–32] Similarly, it has been shown with racial minority groups that exposure to colleagues and peers from those underrepresented backgrounds is likely to result in a higher positive attitude and willingness to care for patients from these backgrounds.[33] This has even been shown in fields outside of medicine, where the more diverse teams were shown to have higher levels of innovation and performance compared with less diverse teams.[34] Through exposure, diversity facilitates the breaking down of stereotypes and barriers. It is only logical that the TGD experience be incorporated into the DEI programs at a medical training level.

WHAT TO INCLUDE IN A TRAINEE DIVERSITY, EQUITY, AND INCLUSION CURRICULUM: THE BASICS

In addition to addressing the role of implicit and explicit bias against TGD individuals, as well as, the pervasive microaggressions and discrimination they face, there are nuance details that should be incorporated into any DEI or cultural competency program. When it comes to gender diversity it is first important to distinguish and define the appropriate language to use. Accepted terminology has changed over time and will continue to change. It is important to remain flexible, patient, and informed. There is a difference between a person's sex, gender identity, and sexual orientation.

- *Sex* refers to one's physical body based on anatomy, hormones, and genetic make-up.[35] Sex is rooted in a binary system, generally either female or male. Current preferred terminology refers to a person's "sex assigned at birth," that is, "assigned male at birth" or "assigned female at birth."
- *Gender identity* refers to how someone identifies in terms of behavior, experience, and personality. Gender identity can be a spectrum rather than a-binary construct.[35]
- *Gender presentation* refers to how one dresses or appears; people may or may not conform to various stereotypical gendered expectations regarding things such as facial hair, make up, and clothing.
- *Transgender* specifically refers to those whose gender identity is discordant with their assigned sex at birth, and
- *Cisgender* refers to those whose gender identity is concordant with their assigned sex at birth.[36]

Some patients identify as neither male or female or both and consider themselves nonbinary or gender nonconforming.

The term *transsexual* has fallen out of favor and should be avoided. This should be distinguished from sexual orientation.

- *Sexual orientation,* which refers to sexual attraction or desires based on an enduring pattern of behavior and is completely independent from gender identity, but also exists on a spectrum.[35]
- *Transition* refers to the process a person may choose to undertake to adjust to their gender identity. Transitioning can occur at any time and can look different for each individual including social presentation, dress, mannerisms, hormone usage, and choice to undergo surgery.[37] Some may choose to participate in some behaviors more than others, or not at all.

The World Professional Association for Transgender Health (WPATH) has published Standards of Care (SOC) guidelines for what should be the approach to optimal care of the TGD community.[38] This includes establishing patients' identity (transgender/cisgender/gender non-conforming/ etc.) and using patients' correct pronouns. Name and pronouns are an important component of one's identity. During one's transition, one may change their name and pronouns to one that better suits their identity. This may differ from the name and pronouns they are given at birth or their legal name. This is referred to as the *chosen name*. One's chosen name is the name individuals prefer to be called by and should be the name used and displayed in a health care setting. The *dead name* is an individual's formal name that they do not give permission to use and should be avoided in both communication and documentation as it is often distressing to patients to be called by or referred to a name that is associated with something that does not align with their identity.[39] Pronouns cannot be assumed based on one's gender identity or name and should be confirmed by *asking* the individual and then documenting appropriately. This may include terminology that differs from the common binary language of "she" and "he" and should be respected. Using the correct pronoun is a way of demonstrating your affirmation of their existence. It is important to employ the correct usage of pronouns for *everyone* and not just exclusively the TGD population given that we all use pronouns so as not to further isolate this community.[39,40] It is recommended providers introduce themselves by name and pronoun followed by asking the patient their name and pronoun in order to standardize and normalize this practice. Lastly, avoid the use of gender-specific honorifics such as Mr and Ms. As this also can result in unnecessary assumptions.[38,39] If in doubt, use the patient's first name to address or refer to them. If you misgender someone by mistake, acknowledge, apologize, then move on.

WHAT TO INCLUDE IN A TRAINEE DIVERSITY, EQUITY, AND INCLUSION CURRICULUM: SETTING THE ENVIRONMENT

Among the WPATH SOC guidelines recommendations for optimal care is the importance for understanding patients' needs and goals and creating an inclusive environment. Aryanpour and colleagues[41] published recommended principles for how to go about applying a gender affirming approach. These basic principles can be applied in almost any health care setting, and it is an easy foundation to begin to incorporate into everyday workplace behavior while fostering a comfortable environment in which TGD patients would want to seek care. Their publication includes recommendations such as the use of gender-diverse or neutral imagery, so that you are not isolating or neglecting any one particular group, using inclusive language on intake forms and when speaking about anatomy, using appropriate pronouns and chosen names, avoiding unrelated invasive questions, and learning and apologizing for any mistakes.

Providers must make special efforts to build rapport and trust with their patients in order to maintain patient safety and achieve desired health outcomes.[42] One suggested approach has been the *trauma-informed care (TIC)* approach. Recognize that TGD patients have a high chance of suffering the effects of trauma and tailor the system to accommodate their needs. The TIC approach provides strategies for breaking down barriers and building a trusting relationship.[43]

1. At the core is patient-centered communication which includes asking about patient's priorities, comforts, and feedback.[43,44]
2. The second step is understanding the health effects of trauma such as an unwillingness to participate in a physical examination or comply with treatment recommendations. Interprofessional, multidisciplinary collaboration can be helpful.
3. Finally, one must be aware of their own biases they bring to the encounter. Providers should be conscientious with words and intentions to avoid further traumatizing patients and being seen as an additional barrier.

WHAT TO INCLUDE IN A TRAINEE DIVERSITY, EQUITY, AND INCLUSION CURRICULUM: COMMUNITY ENGAGEMENT

One does not begin to understand what they *think* they know about another culture and must seek the consultation from the individuals that are directly impacted. Cannon et al[3], in their proposal for better equity in urology, recommended the following community engagement efforts to create a more equitable culture: task force and committees, interest groups and societies, advocacy, and community driven curriculum. Community engagement permits a direct understanding of the community's needs. There are a multitude of ways of incorporating community engagement into a DEI curriculum including working with local LGBTQ + support and interest groups on campus, inviting guest speakers from the community, and consulting local resources such as sexual and gender minority health centers. It is important to be open to feedback and criticism from community members, and above all else *listen*. Learn what is impacting the community and brainstorm ways to best incorporate these practices such as

changing intake forms, having pronouns visible on badges, and ensuring name bracelets accurately reflect correct name and pronoun.

As mentioned earlier, representation and exposure are critical to learning from and understanding another culture and has been shown to increase comfort with caring for patients from that background. An imbalance of workforce representation can perpetuate disparities.[3] It is well known that diversity of racial groups and different sexes are poorly reflected in urology.[45] Although exact numbers have not been reported, there is almost undoubtedly a negligible presence of TGD individuals among urologic students and trainees. Research has shown that patients from underrepresented racial minorities are likely to experience health benefits such as increased shared decision making and decreased mortality when cared for by a racially concordant physician.[30,46] The same can apply to the TGD community. Hence, efforts should be made to enhance recruitment of members of the TGD community within the medical field.

SUMMARY

When it comes to enhancing the field of urology it is important to reflect on the impact our care has on our patients. Among underrepresented minorities, there is a disproportionate incidence of health disparities including the transgender and gender diverse community. Health disparities are rooted in barriers including systemic injustices, patient-related historical trauma, and provider miseducation and bias. As urologists and genitourinary specialists, it is imperative that we become comfortable with how to care for TGD patients. In recent years, the Graduate Medical Education office, American Urologic Association, and American Board of Urology have made more of a concerted effort to correct these injustices in other underrepresented communities and only have begun to extend that to the LGBTQ + community.[47–49] There is an opportunity for urologic programs to address systemic and provider driven barriers at the institutional level through the incorporation of TGD focused, comprehensive DEI, and cultural competency programs. It is not sufficient merely to just educate or introduce these concepts, these are concepts that must be reinforced, understood, and practiced, regardless of one's own beliefs. In the words of Andreja Pejic, a trans-identifying celebrity, "All human beings deserve equal treatment no matter their gender identity or sexuality. To be perceived as what you say you are [and not have that impact how you are treated] is a basic human right."

CLINICS CARE POINTS

- Be aware of knowledge gaps, system break-downs, and personal bias.
- Familiarize yourself with historical context of the trans and gender diverse community.
- Identify and use appropriate language, documentation, and affirming principles.
- Engage the TGD community when developing DEI curriculum; representation matters.
- Do not fear change.

DISCLOSURE

The author has nothing to disclose.

REFERENCES

1. Smith ZL, Eggener SE, Murphy AB. African-american prostate cancer disparities. Curr Urol Rep 2017;18(10):81.
2. Crivelli JJ, Maalouf NM, Paiste HJ, et al. Disparities in kidney stone disease: a scoping review. J Urol 2021;206(3):517–25.
3. Cannon S, Seideman CA, Thavaseelan S, et al. Urologists for equity: a collective approach toward diversity, equity, and inclusion in urology. Urology 2022; 162:33–7.
4. Flores AR, Herman JL, Gates GJ, et al. How many adults identify as transgender in the United States? University of California Los Angeles Williams Institute; 2016. Available at: https://williamsinstitute.law.ucla.edu/publications/trans-adults-united-states/.
5. James S, Herman JL, Rankin S, et al. The report of the 2015 U.S. Transgender survey. Washington, DC: National Center for Transgender Equality; 2016.
6. Zeeman L, Sherriff N, Browne K, et al. A review of lesbian, gay, bisexual, trans and intersex (LGBTI) health and healthcare inequalities. Eur J Public Health 2018;29(5):974–80.
7. Casey LS, Reisner SL, Findling MG, et al. Discrimination in the United States: experiences of lesbian, gay, bisexual, transgender, and queer Americans. Health Serv Res 2019;54(Suppl 2):1454–66.
8. Sineath RC, Blasdel G, Dy GW. Addressing urologic health disparities in sexual and gender minority communities through patient-centered outcomes research. Urology 2022;166:66–75.
9. Reisner SL, Poteat T, Keatley J, et al. Global health burden and needs of transgender populations: a review. Lancet 2016;388(10042):412–36.
10. Chung PH, Spigner S, Swaminathan V, et al. Perspectives and experiences of transgender and non-binary individuals on seeking urological care. Urology 2021;148:47–52.
11. Harrison J, Grant J, Herman JL. A gender not listed here: genderqueers, gender rebels, and otherwise in the national transgender discrimination survey. LGBTQ Policy Journal at the Harvard Kennedy School 2012;2(1):13.
12. Safer JD, Coleman E, Feldman J, et al. Barriers to healthcare for transgender individuals. Curr Opin Endocrinol Diabetes Obes 2016;23(2): 168–71.
13. Allison MK, Marshall SA, Stewart G, et al. Experiences of transgender and gender nonbinary patients in the emergency department and recommendations for health care policy, education, and practice. The J Emerg Medicine 2021;61(4): 396–405.
14. James-Abra S, Tarasoff LA, green d, et al. Trans people's experiences with assisted reproduction services: a qualitative study. Hum Reproduction 2015;30(6):1365–74.
15. 2023 Anti-Trans Legislation Internet. Available at: https://www.tracktranslegislation.com/. Accessed June 6, 2023.
16. 2023 Anti-Trans Bills Tracker Internet. Available at: https://translegislation.com/. Accessed June 6, 2023.
17. Stroumsa D, Shires DA, Richardson CR, et al. Transphobia rather than education predicts provider knowledge of transgender health care. Méd Educ 2019;53(4):398–407.
18. Kent D, Perry K, Vanier C, et al. Assessing comfort of physicians to provide transgender-specific care. Transgender Heal 2022;7(6):533–8.
19. FitzGerald C, Hurst S. Implicit bias in healthcare professionals: a systematic review. BMC Med Ethics 2017;18(1):19.
20. Marcelin JR, Siraj DS, Victor R, et al. The impact of unconscious bias in healthcare: how to recognize and mitigate it. J Infect Dis 2019;220(Supplement_2):S62–73.
21. Haywood C, Lanzkron S, Bediako S, et al. Perceived discrimination, patient trust, and adherence to medical recommendations among persons with sickle cell disease. J Gen Intern Med 2014;29(12): 1657–62.
22. Pellowski JA, Price DM, Allen AM, et al. The differences between medical trust and mistrust and their respective influences on medication beliefs and ART adherence among African-Americans living with HIV. Psychol Heal 2017;32(9):1127–39.
23. Fan Q, Doshi K, Narasimhalu K, et al. Impact of beliefs about medication on the relationship between trust in physician with medication adherence after stroke. Patient Educ Couns 2022;105(4):1025–9.
24. Dubin SN, Nolan IT, Streed CG, et al. Transgender health care: improving medical students' and

residents' training and awareness. Adv Med Educ Pract 2018;9:377–91.

25. Ha M, Ngaage LM, Finkelstein E, et al. P109. Teaching and training in gender-affirming procedures in us academic plastic surgery residency programs. Plastic Reconstr Surg - Global Open. 2022;10(4S):101–2.

26. Burgart JM, Walters RW, Shanahan M. Transgender education experiences among obstetrics and gynecology residents: a national survey. Transgender Heal 2022;7(1):30–5.

27. Morrison SD, Dy GW, Chong HJ, et al. Transgender-related education in plastic surgery and urology residency programs. J Graduate Medical Educ 2017; 9(2):178–83.

28. Social Determinants of Health Internet. Available at: who.int/teams/social-determinants-of-health/equity-and-health. Accessed June 7, 2023.

29. Cooper LA, Roter DL, Johnson RL, et al. Patient-centered communication, ratings of care, and concordance of patient and physician race. Ann Intern Med 2003;139(11):907.

30. Cooper-Patrick L, Gallo JJ, Gonzales JJ, et al. Race, gender, and partnership in the patient-physician relationship. JAMA 1999;282(6):583–9.

31. Komaromy M, Grumbach K, Drake M, et al. The role of black and hispanic physicians in providing health care for underserved populations. N Engl J Med 1996;334(20):1305–10.

32. Betancourt JR, Maina AW. The institute of medicine report "unequal treatment": implications for academic health centers. The Mt Sinai J medicine New York 2004;71(5):314–21.

33. Saha S, Guiton G, Wimmers PF, et al. Student body racial and ethnic composition and diversity-related outcomes in US medical schools. JAMA 2008; 300(10):1135–45.

34. Is There a Payoff from Top-team Diversity? Internet. 2012. Available at: https://www.mckinsey.com/capabilities/people-and-organizational-performance/our-insights/is-there-a-payoff-from-top-team-diversity. Accessed June 7, 2023.

35. Garofalo R. The health of lesbian, gay, bisexual, and transgender people: building a foundation for better understanding. The National Academies Press; 2011.

36. Association AP. Guidelines for psychological practice with transgender and gender nonconforming people. Am Psychol 2015;70(9):832–64.

37. Coleman E, Bockting W, Botzer M, et al. Standards of care for the health of transsexual, transgender, and gender-nonconforming people, version 7. Int J Transgenderism 2012;13(4):165–232.

38. Coleman E, Radix AE, Bouman WP, et al. Standards of care for the health of transgender and gender diverse people, version 8. Int J Transgender Heal 2022;23(S1):S1–259.

39. Transgender Internet. GLAAD Media Reference Guide 11th Edition. Available at: https://www.glaad.org/reference/transgender. Accessed June 4, 2023.

40. Wamsley L. A Guide to Gender Identity Terms Internet. 2021. Available at: https://www.npr.org/2021/06/02/996319297/gender-identity-pronouns-expression-guide-lgbtq#questions. Accessed June 4, 2023.

41. Aryanpour Z, Hubert J, Peters BR. Ten community-informed principles for plastic surgeons beginning gender-affirming care. Plast Reconstr Surg 2023; 151(2). 358e–60e.

42. Pellegrini CA. Trust: the keystone of the patient-physician relationship. J Am Coll Surg 2017;224(2): 95–102.

43. Raja S, Hasnain M, Hoersch M, et al. Trauma informed care in medicine. Fam Community Health 2015;38(3):216–26.

44. Administration SA and MHS. SAMHSA's Concept of Trauma Guidelines and Guidance for a Trauma-INformed Approach. 2014.

45. Winer AG, Hyacinthe LM, Weiss JP, et al. Diversity, equity, and inclusion: advancing curricular development and recruitment. Curr Urol Rep 2023;24(4): 201–4.

46. Greenwood BN, Hardeman RR, Huang L, et al. Physician–patient racial concordance and disparities in birthing mortality for newborns. Proc Natl Acad Sci U S A 2020;117(35):21194–200.

47. AUA Announces Diversity and Inclusion Task Force Internet. Available at: https://auanet.mediaroom.com/2020-12-22-AUA-Announces-Diversity-and-Inclusion-Task-Force. Accessed June 8, 2023.

48. Simons ECG, Thavaseelan S, Saigal C, et al. Diversifying graduate medical education & the urology workforce: re-imagining our structures, policies, practices, norms, & values. Urology 2022;162: 128–36.

49. Husmann DA, Terris MK, Lee CT, et al. The American board of urology: in pursuit of diversity, equity, and inclusion. Urology Pract 2021;8(5): 583–8.

Scales for Assessing Male Sexual Function are not Entirely Applicable to Gay and Bisexual Men with Prostate Cancer

Joanna M. Mainwaring, BScHons[a], Tsz Kin Lee, MD[b],
Richard J. Wassersug, PhD[c], Erik Wibowo, PhD[a],*

KEYWORDS

- Prostate cancer • Gay • Bisexual • MSM • Sexual dysfunction • Scale • Relationship

KEY POINTS

- Many scales have been designed for assessing male sexual function.
- These scales predominantly focus on general sexual function and erection.
- They lack questions on behaviors relevant to men-who-have-sex-with-men (MSM), such as anal sex, masturbation, or sexual activities outside of committed relationships.
- The validation samples rarely mention inclusion of MSM, revealing a clear gap in the clinical evaluation tools available for MSM.

INTRODUCTION

Prostate cancer is the most common type of cancer in men.[1] With earlier diagnosis, prognosis is often excellent, which means that any treatment side effects will impair their quality of life (QoL) for a long period.[2]

Sexual dysfunction is common among men after receiving prostate cancer treatment.[3,4] This may present as erectile dysfunction (ED), loss of ejaculation, orgasm changes, and reduced libido.[5–8] These sexual side effects of treatment can have a large QoL influence on both patients[9] and their partners.[10] Furthermore, sexual dysfunction has been noted as the biggest regret men report about receiving prostate cancer treatment.[11]

Men are affected by sexual dysfunction, both inside and outside of relationships,[12] and the effects may be more profound on men-who-have-sex-with-men (MSM) than heterosexual men.[13] The determinants for QoL differ between MSM and heterosexual men[14]; for example, MSM may be more bothered by the loss of ejaculation[15] as well as urinary, hormonal, and bowel changes.[16] Furthermore, they may be limited in their preferred sexual role (insertive or receptive) with sexual dysfunction.[16] For example, ED may restrict them from having insertive sex, particularly for anal sex where a firmer erection is necessary for anal penetration than vaginal penetration.[17,18] Additionally, more MSM are not in an ongoing relationship and are more likely to have causal sexual partner than heterosexual men,[14,15] and they experience reduced confidence when interacting with new or potential partners.[9,14]

[a] Department of Anatomy, University of Otago, Dunedin, New Zealand; [b] British Columbia Cancer, Abbotsford, Canada; [c] Department of Cellular and Physiological Sciences, University of British Columbia, Vancouver, Canada
* Corresponding author. Department of Anatomy, University of Otago, 270 Great King Street, Dunedin, 9016, New Zealand.
E-mail address: erik.wibowo@otago.ac.nz

Urol Clin N Am 50 (2023) 549–561
https://doi.org/10.1016/j.ucl.2023.06.015
0094-0143/23/© 2023 Elsevier Inc. All rights reserved.

Currently, there is no established and well-validated scale that can adequately assess sexual function of MSM. Despite the many scales that can be used to measure male sexual function, the results from validated scales designed mainly for heterosexual men may not reflect the true impact of sexual dysfunction for MSM recovering from prostate cancer treatment.[12] Here we investigate how broadly applicable are the validated scales, which are currently used for measuring sexual function to the MSM population. As noted above, the sexual dysfunction experienced after prostate cancer treatment may bother MSM significantly more than heterosexual men.[13,15,16] Recognizing this diversity in sexual activity and concerns, we review here the limitations of existing scales for assessing sexual dysfunction of MSM.

In this study, we analyzed scales commonly used to assess male sexual function, with the aim of identifying (1) what sexual variables they measure and (2) how relevant they are to MSM. We anticipate that findings from this review can be used to inform future development of a scale for accurately assessing MSM's sexual dysfunction.

METHODS

We searched on Pubmed and Google Scholar for various questionnaires that had been used to assess male sexual function. From these searches, we identified 21 validated questionnaires relating to sexual dysfunction and its influence on QoL. We excluded one scale—EDITS44 (Erectile Dysfunction Inventory of Treatment Satisfaction)[19] because it was designed to measure sexual function following Viagra treatment. We also excluded the Derogatis Interview for Sexual Functioning because the questionnaire is exceptionally long, and some of the terminology in DISF appears outdated.[20] Each of the remaining scales was analyzed for their item content and the population(s) in which they were validated. Items were included in the analysis if they were relevant to sexual function or QoL and were excluded if they were specific to prepubescent sexual characteristics, nocturnal erection, or partner experiences.

Questionnaire items were categorized into 7 domains: general sexual function, sexual desire, erection, ejaculation, orgasm, relationship, and mood. Questions from each scale were sorted into these domains, and the domains were broken down to indicate which specific variable they were investigating (eg, frequency of the behavior, difficulty of the behavior, satisfaction, and communication).

The validation methods for each scale were also analyzed, particularly in terms of the sexual orientation of the population involved in the validation. This was done to determine whether MSM had been part of the sample used in the development and validation process.

Google Scholar was used to determine the popularity of each scale. The number of published articles that had mentioned or used each scale since it was developed was recorded.

RESULTS
Relevance to Men-Who-Have-Sex-with-Men

Of the 21 articles analyzed regarding validation paper population samples (**Table 1**), only one (4.8% of the 21 articles) of them made any mention of including MSM in the validation process.[21] Despite this, that article did not indicate how many MSM participants were included. Of the remaining 21, five articles express a desire to make their questionnaire applicable to more than heterosexual men but do not indicate any such diversity in their population sample demographics for their validation studies. Nine other studies explicitly exclude nonheterosexual men, refer to partners as women, or refer to intercourse only in the context of vaginal penetration. The remaining articles mention neither inclusion nor exclusion of nonheterosexual men.

Sexual Parameters

In total, we reviewed 21 sexual function scales that had been used to assess male sexual function (**Table 2**). General sexual function was the most commonly covered domain with 66 question items from the 21 questionnaires. Following this were erection with 52 items, ejaculation with 22 items, sexual desire with 28 items, relationship with 17 items, and mood with 11 items, and orgasm with only 6 items across all questionnaires. Body image was least covered with 5 items.

The top 3 types of general sexual function variables were related to satisfaction (24 questions), frequency (11 questions), and confidence (11 questions). For the erection domain, the most common were difficulty (10 questions), firmness (9 questions), and confidence, satisfaction , and mood (6 questions). The ejaculation domain most often focused on difficulty (6 questions) and frequency (4 questions), and the sexual desire domain mainly focused on sex drive (11 questions) and frequency (8 questions). Mood domain mostly covered satisfaction and significance (2 questions each), and relationship domain mostly focused on satisfaction (4 questions) and confidence (3 questions). The orgasm domain focused on satisfaction (4 out of 6 questions). Finally, the body image domain mainly focused on confidence and significance (2 questions each).

Table 1
Inclusion of men-who-have-sex-with-men in validation articles for sexual health questionnaires pertaining to erectile dysfunction

Questionnaires	Proportion of MSM in Validation Paper	Comments
SEAR (Self Esteem and Relationship questionnaire)[22]	Not stated	Only specifies respondents with clinically diagnosed ED
QVS (Quality of Sexual Life questionnaire)[22,23]	Not stated	Only specifies volunteer patients with ED
FSHQ (Florida Sexual History Questionnaire)[24]	Not stated	Criteria for impotent was only described as difficulty maintaining erection suitable for vaginal penetration
TSS (Treatment satisfaction scale)[25]	Not stated	Mentions ED patients and their partners, and refers to the men and women in the study
PIED39 (Psychological Impact of Erectile Dysfunction)[26]	Not stated	
ED-EQoL (Erectile Dysfunction Effect on Quality of Life)[27]	None	Specifies heterosexual men
ASEX (Arizona Sexual Experience scale)[28]	Not stated	Claims to be designed for use in heterosexual and homosexual populations. Subjects pool included men and women
MSHQ (Male Sexual Health Questionnaire)[29]	Not stated	States that it does not assume heterosexual intercourse in its items. In sample, just specifies men aged 50 years old and older with urogenital symptoms, with a stable partner (of 12+ months)
EHS (Erection Hardness Score)[30]	Not stated	Refers to intercourse as vaginal in the Introduction Inclusion criteria includes "stable sexual partner" but does not specify sex of partner
BSFI (Brief male sexual function inventory)[31]	Not stated	Aimed to phrase items so that the participant's partner could have been man or woman
SIEDY (Structured interview on Erectile Dysfunction)[32]	Not stated	One of the questions mentions the potential for partners to be men in the notes about scoring
QEQ (Quality of Erection Questionnaire)[33]	Not stated	Participants were currently involved in a sexual relationship
IIEF (International Index of Erectile Function)[34]	Not stated	
TSS (Treatment Satisfaction Scale)[35]	None	Specifies males with female partners
GRISS (Golombok Rust Inventory of Sexual Satisfaction)[36]	None	Specifies designed for heterosexual couples

(continued on next page)

Table 1
(continued)

Questionnaires	Proportion of MSM in Validation Paper	Comments
QOL-MED (Quality of Life specific to Male Erection Difficulties)[37]	None	Excluded if not in a stable heterosexual relationship
EPIC (Expanded Prostate Cancer Index Composite)[38]	Not stated	
EQS (Erection Quality Scale)[21]	Not stated but implies some says effort was made to increase the representation of homosexual men	Make a point to include input from both heterosexual and homosexual men to help their questionnaire be applicable to both populations
CIPE (Chinese Index of Premature Ejaculation)[39]	Not stated	Just states men and their partners, does mention women when referring to the partners sometimes though
QSF (Scale for Quality of Sexual Function)[40]	Not stated	Targets more general features of sexual function, designed to be applicable to more than just heterosexual men, or just men
PRO (Patient-Reported Outcome)[48]	None	Specifies men in long-term heterosexual relationships

Popularity

Fig. 1 shows how many Google Scholar hits each article assessed in this study has, against the year it was first mentioned. The International Index of Erectile Function (IIEF) ranked far above the rest, with more than 15,000 hits, despite sitting mid-range for year published (1997). The EPIC ranked second but far below the IIEF, with 4260 hits. The ASEX was third, with 2230 hits. The rest of the scales assessed had between 9 and 1490 hits. Year published did not seem to largely influence the number of hits, and the most recent questionnaires were published in 2007 (EHS and QEQ). The number of hits for the PRO questionnaire is not included in this figure because the term "PRO" is not specific to this scale and thus searching the term on Google Scholar results in a multitude of irrelevant hits. However, as of July 2023, the original paper for the PRO scale has been cited 560 times.

DISCUSSION

In this article, we assessed the relevance of existing questionnaires for sexual QoL of MSM, by reviewing the scope of questions in existing questionnaires used to assess sexual function in men, and examining the populations used to validate the questionnaires. Some of these questionnaires are used when men experience sexual dysfunction, to measure its severity and impact on QoL. Circumstances for the use of such questionnaires include the side effects from prostate cancer treatment such as ED and reduced sexual desire. These questionnaires are used in practice for men of varying sexual orientations; however, this review suggests that existing questionnaires may not be entirely suitable for assessing the sexual QoL of MSM, for several reasons.

The sexual variables covered by the various questionnaires analyzed focused largely on general sexual function and erections, particularly on satisfaction and confidence. Other domains such as ejaculation, sexual desire, and relationship are less commonly assessed. Orgasm is the least frequently assessed domain in the questionnaires. Erection may be the primary outcome for assessment because many treatments for sexual dysfunction focus on restoring erections rather than maintaining sexual intimacy. Furthermore, erection is a physiologic function and anatomically accessible, can be objectively measured with more commonality between MSM and heterosexual men. However, other domains, such as sexual desire or orgasm, may be more personal and subjective, thus requiring questionnaires dedicated specially for MSM. Ejaculation itself varies

Table 2
Validated questionnaire categorized sexual domain and the type of variable. Questions specific for partner's sexual function is not included in this table. Some of the questionnaires listed here are copyrighted and thus should not be used clinically or in research without permission from the authors.

Sexual Domain	Questionnaire	Questionnaire item	Variable Type
General sexual function	FSHQ	Sexual intercourse with partner occurs [from never to ≥ twice weekly]	Frequency
		Vaginal penetration with intercourse occurs [from never to always]	Frequency
		When was the last time you and your partner had intercourse?	Frequency
		Masturbation without sexual intercourse occurs [from never to ≥ twice weekly].	Frequency
	GRISS	Do you have sexual intercourse more than twice a week?	Frequency
		Do you find it hard to tell your partner what you like or dislike about your sexual relationship?	Communication
		Are you dissatisfied with the amount of variety in your sex life with your partner?	Satisfaction
		Do you ask your partner what she likes and dislikes about your sexual relationship?	Communication
		Are there weeks in which you do not have sex at all?	Frequency
		Do you enjoy mutual masturbation with your partner?	Satisfaction
		If you want sex with your partner, do you take the initiative?	Confidence
		Do you dislike being cuddled and caressed by your partner?	Satisfaction
		Do you dislike stroking and caressing your partner's genitals?	Satisfaction
		Do you become tense and anxious when your partner wants to have sex?	Anxiety
		Do you enjoy having sexual intercourse with your partner?	Enjoyment
		Do you have sexual intercourse as often as you would like?	Frequency
		Do you refuse to have sex with your partner?	Avoidance
		Do you enjoy cuddling and caressing your partner's body?	Satisfaction
		Do you have feelings of disgust about what you and your partner do during lovemaking?	Satisfaction
		Do you enjoy having your penis stroked and caressed by your partner?	Satisfaction
		Do you try to avoid having sex with your partner?	Avoidance
		Do you find your sexual relationship with your partner satisfactory?	Satisfaction
	SEAR	I felt relaxed about initiating sex with my partner.	Initiation
		I was satisfied with my sexual performance.	Satisfaction
		I felt that sex could be spontaneous.	Initiation
		I was likely to initiate sex.	Initiation
		I felt confident about performing sexually.	Confidence
		I was satisfied with our sex life.	Satisfaction
	PIED39	During the past 4 weeks, my erectile dysfunction makes me feel like less of a man.	Body image
		During the past 4 weeks, my erectile dysfunction makes me feel sexually unattractive.	Body image
		During the past 4 weeks, sex feels like it is not worth the effort.	Satisfaction
		During the past 4 weeks, I feel like something is missing from my sex life if I cannot have intercourse.	Satisfaction
	QoLMED	I have lost confidence in my sexual ability.	Confidence
		I worry about the future of my sex life.	Confidence
		I try to avoid having sex.	Drive
		I am afraid to make the first move toward sex.	Confidence
	EDEQoL	Do you feel less desirable because of your erectile difficulties?	Body image
	QVS	Concerning the pleasure you can reach in your sexuality, you think things are going [very badly - > very well] and in your life you consider this to be [unimportant - > extremely important].	Satisfaction
		Concerning how you feel before starting a sexual activity, you think things are going [very badly - > very well] and in your life you consider this to be [unimportant - > extremely important].	Initiation
			Confidence

(continued on next page)

Table 2
(continued)

Sexual Domain	Questionnaire	Questionnaire item	Variable Type
	TSS	Concerning how sexually normal you feel, you think things are going [very badly - > very well] and in your life you consider this to be [unimportant - > extremely important].	
		During the past 4 weeks, how much pleasure did you get from your sexual activity? (question repeated when on medication too)	Satisfaction
		During the past 4 weeks, how confident did you feel about initiating sex? (question repeated when on medication too)	Confidence
		During the past 4 weeks, how confident were you that you could complete your sexual activity? (question repeated when on medication too)	Confidence
	CIPE	Can you prolong the intercourse time?	Confidence
		[How would you rate] your sexual satisfaction?	Satisfaction
		How about [rating] your confidence in completing sexual activity?	Confidence
		Do you feel anxiety, depression, or stress in sexual activity?	Mood
	PRO	Over the past month, was your satisfaction with sexual intercourse [very poor - > very good]?	Satisfaction
	BSFI	Overall, during the past 30 days, how satisfied have you been with your sex life?	Satisfaction
	MSHQ	Generally, how satisfied are you with the quality of the sex life you have with your main partner?	Satisfaction
		Generally, how satisfied are you with the way you and your main partner show affection during sex?	Satisfaction
		In the last month, how often have you had sexual activity, including masturbating, intercourse, oral sex, or any other type of sex?	Frequency
		Compared with *1 month ago*, has the number of times you have had sexual activity increased or decreased?	Frequency
		In the last month, have you been bothered by these changes in the number of times you have had sexual activity?	Problem
	IIEF	How many times have you attempted sexual intercourse?	Frequency
		How much have you enjoyed sexual intercourse?	Satisfaction
		How satisfied have you been with your overall sex life?	Satisfaction
		How satisfied have you been with your sexual relationship with your partner	Satisfaction
		When you attempted sexual intercourse, how often was it satisfactory for you?	Satisfaction
	QSF	Do you personally experience pain or other problems during sexual intercourse?	Problem
		Do you frequently do sexual self-satisfaction (masturbation)?	Frequency
		Do you occasionally refuse sexual intercourse with your partner, although desired?	Avoidance
		Do your sexual organs respond to sexual desires or dreams as usual?	Ability
		Do you take the initiative to have sexual intercourse with your partner?	Confidence
		Are you happy with your state of excitement before and during sexual intercourse?	Satisfaction
		Does sexuality play an important role in your life?	Significance
Sexual desire	BSFI	During the past 30 days, on how many days have you felt sexual drive?	Frequency
		During the past 30 days, how would you rate your level of sexual drive?	Strength
		In the past 30 days, to what extent have you considered a lack of sex drive to be a problem?	Problem
	FSHQ	How frequently do you think about sexual intercourse?	Frequency
		How frequently would you like to have sexual intercourse?	Frequency
	GRISS	Do you become easily sexually aroused?	Ability
		Do you feel uninterested in sex?	Interest

(continued on next page)

Table 2
(continued)

Sexual Domain	Questionnaire	Questionnaire item	Variable Type
	ASEX	How strong is your sex drive?	Drive
		How easily are you sexually aroused?	Ability
	PIED39	During the past 4 weeks when I cannot have intercourse, I do not feel like having any sex at all.	Drive
		During the past 4 weeks, I avoid sexual opportunities.	Avoidance
	QVS	Concerning your sexual desire, you think things are going [very badly - > very well] and in your life you consider this to be [unimportant - > extremely important].	Drive
	CIPE	[How would you rate] your sexual libido or interest?	Drive
	SIEDY	Did you have more or less desire to make love in the last 3 mo?	Drive
	MSHQ	Generally, how satisfied are you with the number of times you and your main partner have sex?	Satisfaction
		In the last month, how often have you felt an urge or desire to have sex with your main partner?	Drive
		In the last month, how would you rate your urge or desire to have sex with your main partner?	Drive
		In the last month, have you been bothered by your level of sexual desire?	Problem
		Compared with *1 month ago*, has your urge or desire for sex with your main partner increased or decreased?	Drive
	IIEF	How often have you felt sexual desire?	Frequency
		How would you rate your level of sexual desire?	Drive
	QSF	Would you like to have sexual contacts more often?	Frequency
		Does your partner wish for sexual intercourse more often than you do?	Frequency
		Does your partner wish for sexual intercourse less often than you do?	Frequency
		Has your desire for sexual activity (sexual intercourse or masturbation) *de*creased?	Drive
		Has your desire for sexual activity (sexual intercourse or masturbation) *in*creased?	Drive
		Do you often have sexual dreams, fantasies, or desires?	Frequency
		Do you experience great sexual excitement before and during sexual intercourse?	Interest
Erection	BSFI	During the past 30 days, how often have you had partial or full sexual erections when you were sexually stimulated in any way?	Frequency
		During the past 30 days, when you had erections, how often were they firm enough to have sexual intercourse?	Hardness
		How much difficulty did you have getting an erection during the past 30 days?	Difficulty
		In the past 30 days, to what extent have you considered your ability to get and keep erections to be a problem?	Problem
		Difficulty in obtaining an erection for sexual intercourse occurs [from always to never]	Difficulty
		Difficulty in maintaining an erection for sexual intercourse before ejaculation occurs [from always to never].	Difficulty
		Please rate the firmness and rigidity of penile erection before intercourse or masturbation: [never to always].	Firmness
	GRISS	Do you fail to get an erection?	Difficulty
		Do you lose your erection during intercourse?	Difficulty
		Do you get an erection during foreplay with your partner?	Frequency
	QEQ	You had erections hard enough for penetration of your partner [frequency]?	Firmness/frequency
		Your ability to keep your erection to completion of sexual intercourse was [satisfaction rating].	Satisfaction
		The length of time (from when you started sexual activity) until your erection was hard enough to participate in sexual intercourse was [satisfaction rating].	Difficulty
		The length of time you were able to be erect during intercourse was [satisfaction rating].	Duration
		The hardness of your erection was [satisfaction rating].	Firmness
		The overall quality of your erection was [satisfaction rating].	Satisfaction

(continued on next page)

Table 2
(continued)

Sexual Domain	Questionnaire	Questionnaire item	Variable Type
	ASEX	Can you easily get and keep an erection?	Difficulty
	SEAR	I felt confident that during sex my erection would last long enough.	Confidence
	PIED39	During the past 4 weeks when I have trouble with my erection, I feel disgusted by my penis.	Body image
	EDEQoL	Does your inability to have an erection with your partner make you feel guilty?	Confidence
		Does the fact that you are unable to have an erection make you feel like less of a man?	Body image
		Do you feel angry or bitter that you cannot have an erection?	Mood
		Is your sense of identity altered by your lack of erectile function?	Body image
	QoLMED	I feel frustrated because of my erection problem.	Mood
		My erection problem makes me feel depressed.	Mood
		I feel like less of a man because of my erection problem.	Body image
		I worry that I will not be able to get or keep an erection.	Confidence
		I feel that I have lost control over my erections.	Problem
		I blame myself for my erection problem.	Mood
		I feel angry because of my erection problem.	Mood
		I have lost pleasure in sex because of my erection problem.	Satisfaction
		I am embarrassed about my [erection] problem.	Body image
		I worry about letting her down because of my erection problem.	Confidence
		I worry that I am not satisfying her because of my erection problem.	Confidence
		My erection problem interferes with my daily activities.	Problem
		I feel guilty about my erection problem.	Mood
	TSS	During the past 4 weeks, how easy was it for you to get an erection when stimulated? (question repeated when on medication too)	Difficulty
		During the past 4 weeks, how satisfied were you with the amount of time it took before you could get an erection? (question repeated when on medication too)	Satisfaction
		During the past 4 weeks, how satisfied were you with how long your erections lasted? (question repeated when on medication too)	Satisfaction
		During the past 4 wk, how satisfied were you with the hardness of your erections? (question repeated when on medication too)	Satisfaction/firmness
	CIPE	Do you have erections hard enough for sexual intercourse?	Firmness
		Can you maintain erection to complete sexual intercourse?	Difficulty
	MSHQ	*In the last month*, without using drugs such as Viagra, how often have you been able to get an erection when you wanted to?	Frequency
		In the last month, if you were able to get an erection without using drugs such as Viagra, how often were you able to stay hard as long as you wanted to?	Firmness
		In the last month, if you were able to get an erection, without using drugs such as Viagra, how would you rate the hardness of your erection?	Firmness
	IIEF	How often were you able to get an erection during sexual activity?	Frequency
		During sexual intercourse, how often were you able to maintain your erection after you had penetrated (entered) your partner?	Frequency
		When you had erections with sexual stimulation, how often were your erections hard enough for penetration?	Firmness
		When you attempted sexual intercourse, how often were you able to penetrate (enter) your partner?	Firmness
		During sexual intercourse, how difficult was it to maintain your erection to completion of intercourse?	Difficulty
		How do you rate your confidence that you could get and keep an erection?	Confidence
	EHS	How would you rate the hardness of your erection?	Firmness

(continued on next page)

Table 2
(continued)

Sexual Domain	Questionnaire	Questionnaire item	Variable Type
Ejaculation	BSFI	In the past 30 days, how much difficulty have you had ejaculating when you have been sexually stimulated?	Difficulty
		In the past 30 days, how much did you consider the amount of semen you ejaculate to be a problem for you?	Problem
		In the past 30 days, to what extent have you considered your ejaculation to be a problem?	Problem
	FSHQ	Ejaculation with sexual intercourse occurs [__% of the time].	Frequency
		Ejaculation with masturbation occurs [__% of the time].	Frequency
		The ejaculate volume during intercourse or masturbation is usually [volume options from nonexistent to >half teaspoon].	Volume
		The semen ejaculate during intercourse or masturbation is usually [consistency options from clear and watery to yellow thick mucus]	Consistency
	GRISS	Are you able to delay ejaculation during intercourse if you think you may be coming too quickly?	Difficulty
		Can you avoid ejaculating too quickly during intercourse?	Difficulty
	QVS	Concerning the quality of your ejaculation, you think things are going [very badly - > very well] and in your life you consider this to be [unimportant - > extremely important].	Satisfaction
	CIPE	How long from intromission to ejaculation?	Latency
	PRO	Over the past month, was your control over ejaculation during sexual intercourse [very poor -> very good]?	Difficulty
		Over the past month, the severity of my premature ejaculation problem was [severe -> none]?	Difficulty
	SIEDY	Did you notice a reduction of the quantity of the volume of ejaculate?	Volume
	MSHQ	*In the last month*, how often have you been able to ejaculate when having sexual activity?	Frequency
		In the last month, when having sexual activity, how often did you feel that you took too long to ejaculate or "cum"?	Difficulty
		In the last month, when having sexual activity, how often have you felt like you were ejaculating (cumming) but no fluid came out?	Volume
		In the last month, how would you rate the strength or force of your ejaculation?	Force
		In the last month, how would you rate the amount or volume of semen when you ejaculate?	Volume
		Compared with 1 month ago, would you say the physical pleasure you feel when you ejaculate has [increased a lot -> decreased a lot].	Satisfaction
		In the last month, have you experienced any physical pain or discomfort when you ejaculated?	Pain
	IIEF	When you had sexual stimulation or intercourse, how often did you ejaculate?	Frequency
Orgasm	ASEX	How easily can you reach orgasm?	Difficulty
		Are your orgasms satisfying?	Satisfaction
	QVS	Concerning the intensity of your orgasms, you think things are going [very badly - > very well] and in your life you consider this to be [unimportant - > extremely important].	Satisfaction
	TSS	During the past 4 weeks, how satisfied were you with your orgasms?	Satisfaction
	IIEF	When you had sexual stimulation or intercourse, how often did you have the feeling of orgasm or climax?	Frequency
	QSF	Do you reach full satisfaction during sexual activities (orgasm)?	Satisfaction
Mood	PIED39	Do you feel sad or tearful because of your erection difficulties?	Emotion
	QoLMED	I feel different from other men because of my erection problems.	Body image
		I worry about being humiliated because of my [erection] problem.	Confidence
		I get less enjoyment out of life because of my erection problem.	Satisfaction

(continued on next page)

Table 2
(continued)

Sexual Domain	Questionnaire	Questionnaire item	Variable Type
	QVS	Concerning your mood, you think things are going [very badly - > very well] and in your life you consider this to be [unimportant - > extremely important].	Significance
		If you were to live that way for the rest of your life, how satisfied would you be? [very dissatisfied - > very satisfied].	Satisfaction
	MSHQ	*In the last month*, if you have had difficulty getting hard or staying hard without using drugs such as Viagra, have you been bothered by this problem?	Mood
		In the last month, if you have had any ejaculation difficulties or have been unable to ejaculate, have you been bothered by this?	Problem
	PIED39	During the past 4 weeks at times, I have felt so devastated by the performance of my penis that I wanted to die.	Dissatisfaction
	EDEQoL	Are you preoccupied by your erection problems?	Problem
	QSF	Are you yourself unhappy with your common sexual life?	Significance
Body Image	PIED39	During the past 4 weeks, I lack masculine confidence.	Confidence
		During the past 4 weeks, I feel proud of my penis.	Pride
		Is your self-esteem damaged by your erectile problems?	Confidence
	QVS	Concerning your feelings of manliness, you think things are going [very badly - > very well] and in your life you consider this to be [unimportant - > extremely important].	Significance
		Concerning how you feel about yourself, you think things are going [very badly - > very well] and in your life you consider this to be [unimportant - > extremely important].	Significance
Relationship	PIED39	During the past 4 weeks, I feel I could not sustain a new relationship because of my erectile dysfunction.	Confidence
		During the past 4 weeks, my frustration over my erectile dysfunction has a negative effect on my sexual relationship(s).	Problem
		During the past 4 weeks, I am afraid to touch my partner in ways that will make her want to have sex with me.	Confidence
	EDEQoL	Do you feel hurt by your partner's response to your erectile difficulties?	Partner
		Do you feel like a failure because of your erection difficulties?	Confidence
		Are you worried that your erectile problems have affected the closeness between you are your partner?	Partner
	QolMED	I worry that we are growing apart because of my erection problem.	Intimacy
	SIEDY	Do you have other sexual relationships (with people other than your usual partner)?	Partner(s)
	FSHQ	Overall, how satisfactory is your sexual relationship to you?	Satisfaction
	MSHQ	Generally, how satisfied are you with the overall sexual relationship you have with your main partner?	Satisfaction
		Generally, how satisfied are you with the way you and your main partner communicate about sex?	Communication
		Aside from your sexual relationship, how satisfied are you with all other aspects of the relationship you have with your main partner?	Satisfaction
	GRISS	Do you feel there is a lack of love and affection in your sexual relationship with your partner?	Intimacy
	SEAR	I was satisfied with our relationship in general.	Satisfaction
	QSF	Did you have a partner for sexual relations last month?	Partner
		For how long have you been intimate with your current partner?	Partner

between individuals[41,42] and the amount may be especially low in the case of prostate cancer patients because patients will have diminished ejaculation regardless of treatment type. Additionally, orgasm may occur independent of ejaculation, such as in some men after prostatectomy, on ejaculation-inhibiting drugs, after spinal cord injuries, or having diabetes.[5]

The assessed questionnaires provide good insight into general sexual function and

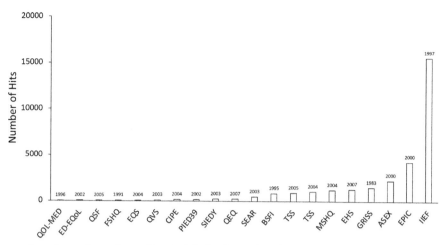

Fig. 1. The number of search results on Google Scholar for each scale and the first year each was validated. The one with the most hits is the IIEF,[34] which is used more often than the rest. The next is EPIC,[38] which is at 4260, followed by ASEX [28] at 2230.

satisfaction. They analyze erection hardness, presence of ejaculation, and presence/experience of orgasm. However, they did lack questions specific to MSM like being a receptive or insertive partner in anal sex. Most items on penetrative sex were related to vaginal penetrative sex. These can not be used as an accurate measure of sexual function for MSM because anal penetration requires firmer erection than vaginal penetration.[17,18] Additionally, masturbation is not commonly covered. Solo/partnered masturbation is more frequently done by MSM than heterosexual men,[43] and hence is an important measure of sexual function for MSM. Furthermore, MSM may have preference to be the insertive or receptive sexual partner.[44] Topics such as anodyspareunia are not discussed but may be experienced by MSM,[45] especially after radiation therapy where receptive partners may have rectal bleeding or sensitivity.[17] Casual sex partnerships (eg, hookups, friends-with-benefits) is also not assessed outside of the QSF but are more common among gay and bisexual men,[46] and MSM with prostate cancer are less likely to be in a monogamous relationship than heterosexual men with prostate cancer.[14,15]

The absence of MSM in almost all validation studies for questionnaires used to measure male sexual function is concerning as these questionnaires appear relevant to heterosexual men but not MSM. Thus, in clinical setting or clinical studies on rehabilitation of sexual dysfunction after prostate cancer treatment, these scales may not adequately capture data meaningful to MSM.

An additional problem with these questionnaires is when men in long-term relationship were included, they were heterosexual couple only. By excluding relationship of MSM and other sexual orientation, which has different dynamics, this may limit the applicability of the questionnaires for population suffered from sexual dysfunction other than heterosexual men.

Given these problems, we have been developing the COMPASS questionnaire for assessing sexual function of MSM. COMPASS addresses additional domains not covered by existing questionnaires reviewed in this study, such as sexual confidence and frequency of various activities or symptoms. In addition, it has items focusing on sexual practices relevant to MSM, such as penetrative/receptive anal sex, solo/partnered masturbation, and regular/casual sexual relationship.

SUMMARY

Validated questionnaires, published to date, are not particularly applicable to assess the sexual QoL of men whose sexual interests and practices go beyond vaginal penetration, such as the MSM community. Sexual domains that are relevant to MSM are largely not assessed by the instruments we reviewed, including domains such as anal sex, masturbation, and casual relationships (which are more common among MSM than heterosexual men). A questionnaire that is specific for measuring sexual function of MSM with prostate cancer is warranted. Such a tool will have an important clinical application for the population and can be used for investigating the outcomes of treatment of sexual dysfunction in men who engage in behavior beyond vaginal penetration.

CLINICS CARE POINTS

- In sum, existing questionnaires designed to assess male sexual function are of limited relevance to MSM. This suggests that a new assessment tool that can capture data relevant to MSM is warranted.

- These questionnaires do not address the sexual function of MSM.

- In this regard, we have been developing the COMPASS questionnaire[9,12,47] to fill gaps in the available questionnaires for assessing male sexual function.

- The COMPASS questionnaire will have clinical and research value for understanding how sexual dysfunction influences sexual QoL of MSM with prostate cancer.

FUNDING

None.

CONFLICT OF INTEREST

None.

REFERENCES

1. American Cancer Society. Key Statistics for Prostate Cancer. 2023; cancer.org/cancer/prostate-cancer/about/key-statistics.html. Accessed 12 April 2023.

2. Downing A, Wright P, Hounsome L, et al. Quality of life in men living with advanced and localised prostate cancer in the UK: a population-based study. Lancet Oncol 2019;20(3):436–47.

3. Kinnaird W, Konteti VKS, Mitra A, et al. Sexual dysfunction in men with advanced prostate cancer. Trend Urol Mens Heal 2021;12(3):7–12.

4. Kinnaird W, Kirby MG, Mitra A, et al. The management of sexual dysfunction resulting from radiotherapy and androgen deprivation therapy to treat prostate cancer: a comparison of uro-oncology practice according to disease stage. Int J Clin Pract 2020;75:e13873.

5. Wibowo E, Wassersug RJ. Multiple orgasms in men—What we know so far. Sex Med Rev 2016; 4(2):136–48.

6. Wibowo E, Wassersug RJ, Robinson JW, et al. How are patients with prostate cancer managing androgen deprivation therapy side effects? Clin Genitourin Cancer 2019;17(3):e408–19.

7. Olsson CE, Alsadius D, Pettersson N, et al. Patient-reported sexual toxicity after radiation therapy in long-term prostate cancer survivors. Br J Cancer 2015;113(5):802–8.

8. Boeri L, Capogrosso P, Ventimiglia E, et al. Depressive symptoms and low sexual desire after radical prostatectomy: early and long-term outcomes in a real-life setting. J Urol 2018;199(2):474–80.

9. Lee TK, Handy AB, Kwan W, et al. Impact of prostate cancer treatment on the sexual quality of life for men-who-have-sex-with-men. J Sex Med 2015; 12(12):2378–86.

10. Movsas TZ, Yechieli R, Movsas B, et al. Partner's perspective on long-term sexual dysfunction after prostate cancer treatment. Am J Clin Oncol 2016; 39(3):276–9.

11. Aning JJ, Wassersug RJ, Goldenberg SL. Patient preference and the impact of decision-making aids on prostate cancer treatment choices and post-intervention regret. Curr Oncol 2012;19(Suppl 3):S37–44.

12. Lee TK, Breau RH, Eapen L. Pilot study on quality of life and sexual function in men-who-have-sex-with-men treated for prostate cancer. J Sex Med 2013; 10(8):2094–100.

13. Simon Rosser BR, Hunt SL, Capistrant BD, et al. Understanding prostate cancer in gay, bisexual, and other men who have sex with men and transgender women: a review of the literature. Curr Sex Health Rep 2019;11:430–41.

14. Ussher JM, Perz J, Kellett A, et al. Health-related quality of life, psychological distress, and sexual changes following prostate cancer: a comparison of gay and bisexual men with heterosexual men. J Sex Med 2016;13(3):425–34.

15. Wassersug RJ, Lyons A, Duncan D, et al. Diagnostic and outcome differences between heterosexual and nonheterosexual men treated for prostate cancer. Urology 2013;82(3):565–71.

16. Hart TL, Coon DW, Kowalkowski MA, et al. Changes in sexual roles and quality of life for gay men after prostate cancer: challenges for sexual health providers. J Sex Med 2014;11(9):2308–17.

17. Goldstone SE. The ups and downs of gay sex after prostate cancer treatment. J Gay Lesb Psychother 2005;9(1 & 2):43–55.

18. Ussher JM, Perz J, Rose D, et al. Threat of sexual disqualification: the consequences of erectile dysfunction and other sexual changes for gay and bisexual men with prostate cancer. Arch Sex Behav 2017;46(7):2043–57.

19. Lewis R, Bennett CJ, Borkon WD, et al. Patient and partner satisfaction with Viagra (sildenafil citrate) treatment as determined by the Erectile Dysfunction Inventory of Treatment Satisfaction Questionnaire. Urology 2001;57(5):960–5.

20. Derogatis LR. The derogatis interview for sexual functioning (DISF/DISF-SR): an introductory report. J Sex Marital Ther 1997;23(4):291–304.

21. Wincze J, Rosen R, Carson C, et al. Erection quality scale: initial scale development and validation. Urology 2004;64(2):351–6.

22. Cappelleri JC, Althof SE, Siegel RL, et al. Development and validation of the Self-Esteem And Relationship (SEAR) questionnaire in erectile dysfunction. Int J Impot Res 2004;16(1):30–8.

23. Costa P, Arnould B, Cour F, et al. Quality of Sexual Life Questionnaire (QVS): a reliable, sensitive and reproducible instrument to assess quality of life in subjects with erectile dysfunction. Int J Impot Res 2003;15(3):173–84.

24. Geisser ME, Jefferson TW, Spevak M, et al. Reliability and validity of the Florida Sexual History Questionnaire. J Clin Psychol 1991;47(4):519–28.

25. Kubin M, Trudeau E, Gondek K, et al. Early conceptual and linguistic development of a patient and partner treatment satisfaction scale (TSS) for erectile dysfunction. Eur Urol 2004;46(6):768–74 [discussion: 774-765].

26. Latini DM, Penson DF, Colwell HH, et al. Psychological impact of erectile dysfunction: validation of a new health related quality of life measure for patients with erectile dysfunction. J Urol 2002;168(5):2086–91.

27. MacDonagh R, Ewings P, Porter T. The effect of erectile dysfunction on quality of life: psychometric testing of a new quality of life measure for patients with erectile dysfunction. J Urol 2002;167(1):212–7.

28. McGahuey CA, Gelenberg AJ, Laukes CA, et al. The Arizona Sexual Experience Scale (ASEX): reliability and validity. J Sex Marital Ther 2000;26(1):25–40.

29. Rosen RC, Catania J, Pollack L, et al. Male Sexual Health Questionnaire (MSHQ): Scale development and psychometric validation. Urology 2004;64(4): 777–82.

30. Mulhall JP, Goldstein I, Bushmakin AG, et al. Validation of the erection hardness score. J Sex Med 2007; 4(6):1626–34.

31. O'Leary MP, Fowler FJ, Lenderking WR, et al. A brief male sexual function inventory for urology. Urology 1995;46(5):697–706.

32. Petrone L, Mannucci E, Corona G, et al. Structured interview on erectile dysfunction (SIEDY): a new, multidimensional instrument for quantification of pathogenetic issues on erectile dysfunction. Int J Impot Res 2003;15(3):210–20.

33. Porst H, Gilbert C, Collins S, et al. Development and validation of the quality of erection questionnaire. J Sex Med 2007;4(2):372–81.

34. Rosen RC, Riley A, Wagner G, et al. The international index of erectile function (IIEF): a multidimensional scale for assessment of erectile dysfunction. Urology 1997;49(6):822–30.

35. Rosen R, Goldstein I, Huang XY, et al. The Treatment Satisfaction Scale (TSS) is a sensitive measure of treatment effectiveness for both patients and partners: results of a randomized controlled trial with vardenafil. J Sex Med 2007;4(4 Pt 1):1009–21.

36. Rust J, Golombok S. The GRISS: a psychometric instrument for the assessment of sexual dysfunction. Arch Sex Behav 1986;15(2):157–65.

37. Wagner TH, Patrick DL, McKenna SP, et al. Cross-cultural development of a quality of life measure for men with erection difficulties. Qual Life Res 1996;5(4):443–9.

38. Wei JT, Dunn RL, Litwin MS, et al. Development and validation of the expanded prostate cancer index composite (EPIC) for comprehensive assessment of health-related quality of life in men with prostate cancer. Urology 2000;56(6):899–905.

39. Yuan YM, Xin ZC, Jiang H, et al. Sexual function of premature ejaculation patients assayed with Chinese Index of Premature Ejaculation. Asian J Androl 2004;6(2):121–6.

40. Heinemann LA, Potthoff P, Heinemann K, et al. Scale for Quality of Sexual Function (QSF) as an outcome measure for both genders? J Sex Med 2005;2(1): 82–95.

41. Oshio S, Ashizawa Y, Yotsukura M, et al. Individual variation in semen parameters of healthy young volunteers. Arch Androl 2004;50(6):417–25.

42. Mayorga-Torres BJM, Camargo M, Agarwal A, et al. Influence of ejaculation frequency on seminal parameters. Reprod Biol Endocrinol 2015;13:1–7.

43. Dodge B, Herbenick D, Fu TC, et al. Sexual behaviors of U.S. men by self-identified sexual orientation: results from the 2012 National Survey of Sexual Health and Behavior. J Sex Med 2016;13:637–49.

44. Moskowitz DA, Rieger G, Roloff ME. Tops, bottoms, and versatiles. Sex Relation Thor 2000;23.191–202.

45. Wheldon CW, Bates AJ, Polter EJ, et al. Unrecognized sexual dysfunction in gay and bisexual men after prostate cancer treatment: the antecedents and impact of anodyspareunia. J Sex Med 2023; 20(4):515–24.

46. Herbenick D, Reece M, Schick V, et al. Sexual behavior in the United States: results from a national probability sample of men and women ages 14-94. J Sex Med 2010;7:255–65.

47. Lee TK, Wibowo E, Dowsett GW, et al. Development of a sexual quality of life questionnaire for men-who-have-sex-with-men with prostate cancer. J Sex Med 2022;10:100480.

48. Patrick DL, Althof SE, Pryor JL, et al. Premature ejaculation: an observational study of men and their partners. J Sex Med 2005;2(3):358–67.

Cancer Screening for Transgender Individuals
Guidelines, Best Practices, and a Proposed Care Model

Joshua Sterling, MD, MSc[a], Jeffrey Carbonella, MD[a], Tashzna Jones, MD[a],
Stephanie Hanchuk, MD[a], Paris Kelly, MS[b],
Maurice M. Garcia, MD, MAS[c,d,e,f],*

KEYWORDS

- Cancer screening • Trans male • Trans female • Transgender health
- Gender-affirming hormone therapy • Gender-affirming surgery

KEY POINTS

- Physicians must address the need for transgender patients' cancer screening and for it to be tailored to the individuals' "stage of transition" as it relates to gender-affirming hormone therapy (GAHT), nongenital gender-affirming surgery (GAS), genital GAS, and the degree to which reproductive organs have been surgically removed as this may impact cancer risk.
- Although a theoretic risk can be incurred with the use of GAHT, there are no long-term studies done to show an increased risk of cancer in patients on puberty blockers or long-term GAHT.
- There remain paucity of data in the literature regarding cancer screening in the transgender population and more prospective trials are needed to formalize clear and consistent evidence-based cancer screening guidelines in this population.
- What state of gender transition a patient exists in at any given time affects all biopsychosocial systems, as they relate to cancer and other urologic domains.

INTRODUCTION

Widespread cancer screenings have resulted in improved cancer survival rates over the last 50 years inclusive of a 13% decrease in colorectal cancer mortality and a 14% reduction in lung cancer mortality.[1,2] Mammograms and Pap smears have ameliorated breast and cervical cancer prognoses.[3,4] Decreases in prostate cancer mortality are partially attributable to prostate specific antigen (PSA) screening. The American Cancer Society (ACS), US Preventative Services Task Force (USPSTF), and numerous professional organizations (ACS, American Medical Association [AMA], American Urologic Association [AUA], and American College of Obstetricians and Gynecologists [ACOG]) have recommendations for early cancer detection in average and high-risk cisgender patients. However,

Note: race/ethnicity denotes that both race and ethnicity were combined in this analysis, but that race and ethnicity are distinctly different and not synonymous.

[a] Department of Urology, Yale School of Medicine, New Haven, CT, USA; [b] Quinnipiac University, Hamden, CT, USA; [c] Division of Urology, Cedars-Sinai Medical Center, Los Angeles, CA, USA; [d] Department of Urology, University of California San Francisco, San Francisco, CA, USA; [e] Department of Anatomy, University of California San Francisco, San Francisco, CA, USA; [f] Department of Urology, Cedars-Sinai Transgender Surgery and Health Program, Gender Affirming Genital Surgery and Sexual Medicine, Cedars-Sinai Medical Center, Los Angeles, 8631 West Third Street, Suite 1070W, Los Angeles, CA 90048, USA

* Corresponding author. Department of Urology, Cedars-Sinai Medical Center, Los Angeles, Cedars-Sinai Transgender Surgery and Health Program, Gender Affirming Genital Surgery and Sexual Medicine, 8631 West Third Street, Suite 1070W, Los Angeles, CA 90048.
E-mail address: Maurice.garcia@cshs.org

Urol Clin N Am 50 (2023) 563–576
https://doi.org/10.1016/j.ucl.2023.06.014

guidelines modifications are required to better serve the transgender community.

Currently, the World Professional Association of Transgender Health (WPATH) lacks cancer screening guidelines. Transgender patients' cancer screening must be tailored to the individuals' "stage of transition" as it relates to gender-affirming hormone therapy (GAHT), nongenital and genital gender-affirming surgery (GAS), and current anatomic inventory. The WPATH Standards of Care (SOC) version 8 states, *"We have insufficient evidence to estimate the prevalence of cancer of the breast or reproductive organs among TGD populations... However, cancer screening should commence, in general, according to local guidelines... In caring for transgender patients, the PCP should maintain an updated record of which organs are present in TGD patients so that appropriate, routine screening can be offered."*[5] Databases including the Surveillance, Epidemiology and End Result and National Cancer Databases do not include nonbinary genders, prohibiting estimates of cancer risk in transgender populations. The UK study found gay and bisexual men had an increased likelihood of cancer diagnoses when compared with heterosexual males, although an increased prevalence is due to higher rates of viral-related cancers such as Kaposi's sarcoma, anal cancer, and penile cancer.[6] Investigation in the United States rely on extrapolations of cancer rates in regions with large populations of LGBT individuals[7,8] with varied results and no definitive conclusions.

Increased high-risk behaviors including smoking, alcohol, drug use, obesity along with Human Immunovirus (HIV) rates in the LGBT community are often used to explain the differences in cancer rates when compared with cisgender populations.[9,10] In 2013, 1.9% of HIV tests in transgender individuals were positive compared with 0.9% in cisgender males and 0.2% in cisgender females.[11] The estimated prevalence of HIV among transgender women of reproductive age is 21.7% (95% CI: 18.4%–25.1%), 34 times higher than age-matched cisgender adults.[12,13]

Discrimination and stigmatization against transgender patients reduces the frequency of health care encounters. Transgender individuals have reported difficulties interfacing with the health care system: 19% reported refusal of care, 28% reported harassment, and 50% reported being turned off from health care systems due to the lack of gender nonconforming providers.[14,15] Clinicians may fail to provide the appropriate screening and counseling based on underreporting and lack of discussion surrounding the patient's anatomic inventory.

Our aim is to review the current guidelines and practice patterns of cancer screening in transgender patients and, where evidence-based data are lacking, to draw from cisgender screening guidelines to suggest best practice screening approaches for transgender patients.

We performed a systematic search of PubMed, Google Scholar, and Medline, using all iterations of the following search terms: transgender, gender nonconforming, gender nonbinary, cancer screening, breast cancer, ovarian cancer, uterine cancer, cervical cancer, prostate cancer, colorectal cancer, anal cancer, and all acceptable abbreviations. Given the limited amount of existing literature, inclusion was broad. After eliminating duplicates and abstracts, all queries yielded 85 unique publications. We present the following article in accordance with the Systematic reviews and Meta-Analyses extension for Scoping Reviews (PRISMA-ScR) reporting checklist (available at https://doi.org/10.210337/tau-20-954).

Cancer Screening Guidelines

Early cancer detection has contributed to better health outcomes.[1,3,4] However, when proposing cancer screenings, the advantages of early detection must be weighed against the likelihood of harm due to over treatment. Open, regular communication between patients and physicians is crucial to perform shared decision-making regarding appropriate cancer screenings.

To identify high-risk populations who may benefit from screening, large population-based databases are used. These databases are unsuccessful at capturing transgender and nonbinary people.[16,17] Few recommendations exist for cancer screening designed specifically for transgender people. In this article, all recommendations for screening guidelines were originally designed for cisgender people and applied to the transgender population based on available case series.

Youth Cancer Risk

Gender dysphoria decreases the rate of cancer screenings for birth organs. Up to 71% of patients have their first experiences with gender dysphoria at an early age, between the ages of 3 and 6 years.[18] A routine examination of native organs can exacerbate gender dysphoria. When transgender patients seek out medical attention, the focus is often on mental health or GAHT with little attention to preventative health.[19,20] Traumatizing interactions with health care further decrease the likelihood that conversations around screening will occur. Initiating these conversations can be challenging, especially for youth who are on GAHT.

Providers and patients alike are concerned about the potential effects of GAHT on cancer risk. It is reassuring that GAHT has been shown to be safe in transgender patients and result in predictable hormone levels.[21] Although a theoretic risk can be incurred with the use of GAHT, there are no long-term studies showing an increased risk of cancer in patients on puberty blockers or long-term GAHT[22,23]

Social Transition and Cancer Risk

Throughout the gender transition process, the medical professionals that a patient sees can change which could affect the prioritization of longitudinal cancer screening guidelines. When obtaining birth-sex-based cancer screening, transgender patients report feeling uncomfortable doing so in the acknowledgment that they possess birth-sex anatomy. For instance, transmasculine patients may be less likely to follow up with a gynecologist after initiating GAHT and/or genital GAS, even though they continue to have gynecologic cancer risk factors. According to a 2011 ACOG statement, medical professionals should be able to treat transgender patients or at the very least be able to send them for regular examinations and screenings as necessary.[24]

Gender-Affirming Hormone Therapy and Cancer Risk

For transgender patients on GAHT, the long-term effects remain unknown. No conclusive long-term studies have been conducted to determine the overall effects of these hormones on health or specific cancer risk. The use of long-term GAHT in transgender individuals is unique to this population and is not directly parallel to the use in cisgender individuals. Primarily, the use of GAHT results in elevation of both feminizing and masculinizing hormones before the removal of birth sex gonads. The appropriate doses of hormones for individuals vary widely and can result in potential exposure to high levels of hormones and metabolites, which may alter the risk of sex hormone-sensitive cancers.

The role of sex hormones on breast and prostate cancer has been studied extensively in cisgender patients and is emerging as a research area for the transgender population. In cis individuals, the presence of estrogen and progesterone receptors affects the prognosis and treatment of breast cancer.[25] Androgen receptors are also present in breast cancer and can have either tumor suppressive or proliferative effects.[26] Regardless of the specific sex hormone or cancer, the exact effect of exogenous hormones is unknown.[27]

In the Netherlands,[28,29] long-term studies examined over 2300 transgender patients on GAHT between 1975 and 2011. Three cases of breast cancer were identified—two in transfeminine patients and one in a transmasculine patient. One case of prostate cancer was identified. Both malignancy rates lower than reported in cisgender patients.[28,29]

WPATH SOC v8 states transmasculine patients on testosterone-based GAHT have either no increased risk or inconclusive evidence of increased risk of breast, cervical, ovarian, or uterine cancer.[5] Exogenous testosterone may increase the incidence of abnormal Pap smears.

General Transgender Screening Recommendations and Considerations

No general guidelines for cancer screening have been published for transgender individuals. The recommendations proposed in this publication are adapted from guidelines for cisgender patients and applied to the transgender population based on small case series. The proposed screening procedures should not be applied to any patient without a thorough conversation about their stage of transition, anatomic inventory, and high-risk behaviors. According to the WPATH SOC v8, primary care provider should maintain an updated record of which organs are present in transgender patients such that appropriate, routine screening can be offered. This anatomic inventory should be updated based on surgical history or administration of gender-affirming hormones.[5] Given the paucity of large-scale prospective data to inform decisions, these recommendations are solely meant to encourage open communication between transgender patients and their doctors about which cancer screenings may be beneficial.

Surgeons should discuss future cancer risks with patients after GAS. Patients should be provided with documentation regarding their surgical procedure. Surgical pathology findings, including transplanted organs (intestinal transplant vaginoplasty or skin flap vaginoplasty), should be documented. Physicians should also make note of the organs remaining and council patients on the importance of following existing screening guidelines.[5]

Colon cancer

All patients over the age of 50 years should undergo either a guaiac-based fecal occult blood test, a fecal immunochemical test, a multitarget stool DNA test, a double-contrast barium enema, or a CT colonography to screen for colorectal cancer.[30] Any positive test requires a follow-up colonoscopy. High-risk patients due to a personal or family history of colon cancer or inflammatory bowel disease should follow more rigorous monitoring schedules.[30] No current studies are available to specifically assess colorectal cancer rates in the transgender population. At any stage of transition, transgender people should adhere to these guidelines. Watanabe and colleagues published a case study of a transfeminine patient who underwent robotic low anterior resection for rectal cancer 12 years after vaginoplasty. Only a very thin membrane separates the neovaginal cavity from the bladder and rectum leading to an increased risk of neovaginal injury during surgery. Given this increased risk, patients presenting with colorectal cancer after vaginoplasty should be treated by surgeons who are familiar with their anatomy.[31]

Lung cancer

Annual lung cancer screening with low-dose helical CT should be discussed in current or former smokers of either sex with at least a 30-pack-year smoking history or former smokers who stopped smoking less than 15 years ago.[30] No studies have specifically assessed lung cancer rates in the transgender population. At any stage of transition, all transgender people should adhere to these screening recommendations.

Anal cancer

Specific guidelines for anal cancer screenings are lacking. However, the American Society of Clinical Oncology endorses routine testing for high-risk patients, defined as HIV-infected individuals who engage in anal receptive intercourse. The prevalence of human papillomavirus (HPV) and rate of HPV vaccination within the transgender community is not well reported. The available data categorize all LGBT individuals into a single category which fails to provide specificity. Physicians have been shown to be reluctant to discuss HPV risks or perform routine anal examinations.[32]

Cytology from an anal Pap smear is the most widely used screening method for anal cancer. Confirmatory testing is done with anoscopic biopsy. Cytologic screening is geared toward identifying premalignant anal high-grade squamous intraepithelial lesions.[33] A 2017 study of 22 HIV-positive transfeminine patients showed that 91% of patients who underwent anal biopsies were found to have some degree of dysplasia, even though none of the patients screened were found to have cancer.[33] Furthermore, a study in Thailand reported 42% of transfeminine patients screened had abnormal cytology.[34] Evidence suggests that transfeminine patients, especially HIV-positive patients, are at an increased risk of anal squamous intraepithelial lesions. Consequently, there is a critical need for a standardized, evidence-based screening method. No consensus has been reached, but Thompson and colleagues advise the screening of any transfeminine patients with multiple lifetime sexual partners starting at age 21 years.[35] Transmasculine patients who engage in anal intercourse would benefit from discussing screening options with their physician. These guidelines should be followed regardless of the stage of the patient's transition.

Sex Organ-Specific Screening Recommendations: Patients Assigned Female at Birth

WPATH SOC v8 states that transmasculine patients on testosterone-based GAHT have no increased risk or inconclusive evidence of increased risk of breast, cervical, ovarian, or uterine cancer.[5] Olsen and colleagues reported an increased risk of ovarian cancer in cis-females that used testosterone supplements, but it is difficult to translate these data to the transmasculine population. Appropriate gynecologic follow-up in transmasculine patients is scarce.[36] Grynberg and colleagues performed a histologic analysis of specimens from 112 patients who underwent at least 6 months of GAHT before total hysterectomy and bilateral salpingo-oophorectomy. No cases of ovarian, uterine, or cervical cancer or premalignant changes were observed leading to the conclusion GAHT did not contribute to an increased cancer risk.[37] There are reports of female reproductive organ malignancies in transmasculine patients: six cases of ovarian cancer, three cases of cervical cancer, one case of vaginal cancer, and one case of uterine cancer.

Breast cancer

Breast cancer screening recommendations for cis-females include an annual or biennial mammogram after 50 years.[29,38] Screening may start earlier based on family history or patient preference. Research has shown that transmasculine patients on GAHT do not have an increased risk of breast cancer.[5] Moreover, early reports suggest that the risk is similar to cis-males.[29,38] Data from the Veterans Health Administration found 52% of transmasculine patients had undergone GAHT treatment and identified seven cases of breast cancer in transmasculine patients. Overall incidence was 20/100,000 patients yearly regardless of hormone exposure, which was not higher than the expected rate.[38] Four cases of invasive breast cancer were found in 1229 transmasculine patients; lower than expected compared with cisgender women (incidence ratio 0.2, 95% CI: 0.1–0.5).[39]

Breast cancer screening guidelines are evolving with respect screening age and frequency. In transmasculine patients, the process is further complicated by a limited understanding of effects of GAHT and lack of reliable epidemiologic data. Transmasculine patients who have *NOT* undergone bilateral mastectomy or who have *ONLY* undergone breast reduction should follow screening guidelines for cis-females. However, simply following the guidelines for cisgender females following risk-reducing mastectomy in transgender male patients poses risks. Risk-reduction mastectomy and gender-affirming mastectomy have different aims. In GAS, residual breast tissue prevents an undesirable chest indent, whereas risk-reduction mastectomy removes a substantial amount of breast tissue which limits performance of a mammography. GAS often preserves adequate breast tissue to allow for a mammogram in transgender males. Breast cancer has developed in transgender male patients following GAS mastectomy.[40,41]

No consensus, evidence-based screening guidelines for breast cancer in transgender patients exist. However, recent guidelines were proposed by the American College of Radiology.[42] The risk of breast cancer in transmasculine patients is comparable to the general population regardless of transition stage; thus, existing cancer screening guidelines should be followed.[29,43] Individuals who undergo GAS of the chest should have ongoing breast cancer screening overseen by their primary care physician (PCP) who should stay up-to-date on guidelines as they are subject to change.[5]

Uterine cancer

Little evidence exists to endorse standard screening for uterine and endometrial cancer in cis-females. In transmasculine patients, only 8% have reported the removal of cervix and uterus according to a 2015 survey.[44] Given the lack of standardized screening guidelines, transgender patients should report any abnormal vaginal bleeding and follow generalized recommendations. A single report exists of uterine cancer discovered during preoperative evaluation for GAS[45] in which the patient presented with abnormal bleeding after several years of amenorrhea. Endometrial evaluation is recommended as a standard preoperative care before GAS. Transgender patients are not recommended to undergo routine screening or prophylactic hysterectomies.[45,46]

Cervical cancer

For the cisgender female patient, cervical cancer screening is as follows: starting at 21 year old, the Pap smear should be performed.[30] After age 30 years, HPV DNA tests should be done in concert with Pap smears. Screening should continue until age 66 years and be discontinued after two consecutive negative test or if cervix is surgically absent.[30]

According to one study, 9.2% fewer transmasculine patients were appropriately screened for cervical cancer when compared with cisgender females.[47,48] GAHT has not been found to increase cervical cancer risk. Still, transmasculine patients may have increased risk due to higher active HIV rates.[11–13] HIV infection can lead to persistence of HPV infections, thereby increasing cervical cancer risk. Further research is needed to appreciate the true risk of HPV infection and related cancer risk in the transgender population.[27,49] Screening can be challenging in the transmasculine population due to GAHT effect of atrophy of cervical epithelium. The atrophic cells lead to poor sampling inadequate for testing, approximately $10\times$ higher than cis-females.[50] In addition, use and length of testosterone supplementation along with higher body mass index can be associated with inadequate Pap smear samples.[50] Insufficient Pap smear samples often lead to delays in testing and inappropriate screening intervals.[49] Sampling a wide area, using a variety of sampling equipment, and prescribing topical estrogen for application before Pap smear increases the likelihood of obtaining sufficient samples.

The WPATH SOC v8 recommends that health care professionals offer cervical cancer screening to transgender and gender diverse people who have a cervix aligned with guidelines for cis-women.[5,51] Therefore, if the cervix is present transmasculine patients should undergo Pap smear every 3 years starting at age 21 years. Providers should be cognizant of performing pelvic and speculum examinations to minimize potential physical and emotional trauma and aware of alternatives to speculum examinations and cervical cytology, such as provider- or self-collected high-risk HPV swabs, as these may be of benefit for patients unable to tolerate a pelvic examination.

Ovarian cancer

The USPSTF recommends against routine ovarian cancer screening for cisgender woman.[52] No available evidence suggests that transmasculine patients are at an increased risk of ovarian cancer. Therefore, transmasculine patients should follow the same guidelines as cis-females.[36,53] Prophylactic oophorectomy should not be performed without other identified risk factors.[53]

Vulva cancer

No screening guidelines exist for vulvar cancer for cisgender women. A solitary case of vaginal cancer in a transmasculine patient has been reported in the literature.[54] Routine screening is therefore not recommended.

Sex Organ-Specific Screening Recommendations: Patients Assigned Male at Birth

In addition to exogenous estrogen, GAHT for transfeminine patients may also incorporate Gonadotropoin Releasing Hormone (GnRH) antagonists to halt production of natal sex hormones. The administration of GnRH antagonists further complicates the intricate relationships between sex and cancer risk as there is an unknown impact on sex-specific tumors. To date, research on long-term impact of GAHT on cancer risk is limited, but no evidence exists that GAHT increases cancer risk.[5,55,56]

Testicular cancer

Cis-males should undergo physical examination each year to assess for testicular masses. Two occurrences of testicular cancer in transfeminine patients have been documented; one was discovered incidentally following orchiectomy, and the other was detected due to rising testosterone levels in the setting of feminizing hormone treatment.[57,58] Patients with testicles should undergo yearly physical examinations to assess for testicular masses at any stage of transition.

Prostate cancer

For cis-males, prostate cancer screening recommendation is for patients more than age 50 years to have PSA level checked and undergo digital rectal examination. In high-risk patients—African Americans and patients with a family history of prostate cancer—screening should occur earlier. In transfeminine patients, the risk of prostate cancer is lower than cis-males; however, the risk is not zero.

GAS for transfeminine patients does not routinely include prostatectomy; therefore, it is prudent to continue anatomically appropriate screening. Gooren and colleagues reported 0.04% prostate cancer prevalence in a cohort of 2300 patients; however, these patients did not undergo routing prostate cancer screening; thus, the true prevalence may be higher.[28] Tabaac and colleagues reported that transfeminine patients were less likely to discuss prostate issues or have a PSA test when compared with cis-males.[14] Recent case reports, including 10 cases of prostate cancer in transfeminine patients including 6 that were metastatic on presentation, are challenging the idea that "dissemination of prostate cancer is inhibited by eliminating androgens or neutralizing their effect with the injection of estrogens."[59] In all reported cases of prostate cancer in a transfeminine patient, the use of estrogen was prevalent. Therefore, studies suggest that estrogen may not have a protective effect and may alternatively play a role in the development of prostate cancer.[60,61] In a retrospective cohort study, Rastrelli and colleagues looked at 2967 hypogonadal male patients to establish a relationship between testosterone deficiency and serum PSA levels leading to a PSA cutoff of 0.612 ± 0.022 ng/mL maximized sensitivity and specificity for prostate cancer detection in hypogonadal men.[62] Similar PSA values may be applicable to transfeminine patients; however, further research is necessary to establish evidence-based cutoffs for PSA values and PSA velocities in the transgender population.[63,64] Although the sexual dysfunction after prostate cancer therapy in cisgender men has been explicitly studied,[65] the degree and type of sexual dysfunction experienced by transfeminine patients remains unknown. It is imperative that physicians remain conscious of their unique sexual concerns. The WPATH and Endocrine Society both recommend transfeminine patients follow the present guidelines for prostate cancer screening in cis-males with one notable stipulation—a PSA of 1 ng/mL should be used as the upper limit of normal.[51,66,67]

Penile cancer

In the cisgender community, there are insufficient data to support screening for penile cancer. At present, there are no reported cases of penile cancer in the transgender population.

Breast cancer in males/transmasculine patients

Insufficient evidence exists to support breast cancer screening in cis-males. Brown and colleagues, using data from the Veteran Health Administration, found three cases of breast cancer in transfeminine patients who had undergone GAHT. The overall incidence was 20/100,000 patient yearly regardless of hormone exposure.[38] de Blok and colleagues found 15 cases of breast cancer out of 2260 transfeminine patients reporting a 46-fold increased risk of breast cancer compared with cisgender men.[39] Most tumors presented in a typical female pattern, they were ductal carcinoma and receptor positive.[39]

Transfeminine patients have an overall lifetime exposure to estrogen and progesterone orders of magnitude smaller than cisgender females. The presence of estrogen and progesterone receptors is a major factor in the prognosis and treatment of breast cancer.[25] Androgen receptors can have tumor suppressive or tumor proliferative effects depending on the type of breast cancer. Currently, no evidence suggests that GAHT increases cancer risk, but long-term effects remain unknown.[26,27] Evidence suggests that testosterone is protective

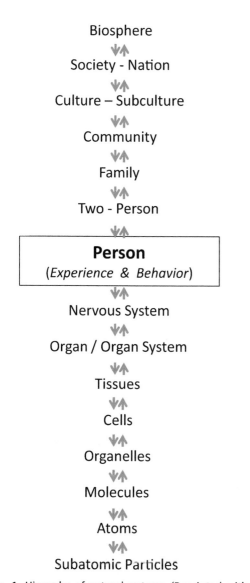

Biosphere

Society - Nation

Culture – Subculture

Community

Family

Two - Person

Person
(*Experience & Behavior*)

Nervous System

Organ / Organ System

Tissues

Cells

Organelles

Molecules

Atoms

Subatomic Particles

Fig. 1. Hierarchy of natural systems. (Reprinted with permission from the American Journal of Psychiatry, Volume 137, Issue 5, "The clinical application of the biopsychosocial model," p. 537 George L. Engel, (Copyright © 1980). American Psychiatric Association. All Rights Reserved.)

and the loss of circulating testosterone combined with an elevation in estrogen levels may lead to an increased risk for transfeminine patients compared with cis-males.[26] Transfeminine patients commonly have dense breasts, which are an independent risk factor for breast cancer and increase the rate of false-negative mammograms.

There are no current data or recommendations on how GAHT affects breast cancer risk for patients with BRCA1 mutations. Only 6% of cisgender men with BRCA1 mutation develop breast cancer compared with 78% of cisgender females.[68]

One case report exists of the management of a transgender female with a BRCA1 mutation. This patient refused prophylactic mastectomy, continued GAHT after her vaginoplasty and bilateral orchiectomy, and is undergoing screening based on guidelines for cisgender women.[69]

Breast cancer screening guidelines are evolving with respect to what age to begin screening and frequency. For transfeminine patients, mammograms are recommended every 2 years in patients more than 50 years who have had 5 to 10 years of GAHT treatment.[68] As recommended in WPATH SOC v8, "We recommend health care professionals follow local breast cancer screening guidelines developed for cisgender women in their care of transgender and gender diverse people who have received estrogens, taking into consideration the length of time of hormone use, dosing, current age, and the age at which hormones were initiated."[5]

Malignancies of the Neovagina

Tissues used to create neovaginas have the potential to develop malignancy. Genital skin flaps are the gold standard for GAS, whereas intestinal transplant vaginoplasty has been classically used for congenital or traumatic absence of the vagina. Intestinal transplant neovaginas can develop adenocarcinoma. Skin flap neovaginas can develop squamous cell carcinoma (SCC). Four cases of neovaginal SCC in transfeminine patients have been reported with HPV infection implicated in three out of four cases.[70] The median age for vaginoplasty was 27 year old with a median latency before the diagnosis of 27 years ranging from 18 to 45 years.[54,70] Seven reported cases of adenocarcinoma after colon transplant vaginoplasty exist; none of these cases were in transgender patients.[71,72]

For causal factors, chemical stimulants and irritants in semen may contribute to malignancies of the neovagina. Grosse and colleagues examined cytology from 20 neovagina washings, 3 colon transplants, and 17 skin grafts, and discovered 30% had abnormal cytology.[73] Thus, the investigators concluded that patients with neovaginas, irrespective of graph tissue, were prone to precancerous lesions and therefore advised patients to follow cancer screening programs.[73–75]

Currently, there are no established guidelines for neovagina cancer screening. Patients who undergo vaginoplasty should receive routine gynecologic examination including speculum and digital examinations to assess for HPV condylomas.[5,76,77] Cytology testing in transgender individuals may be helpful dependent on vaginoplasty tissue.[78] HPV vaccination is recommended for all transgender patients less than age 26 years.[30]

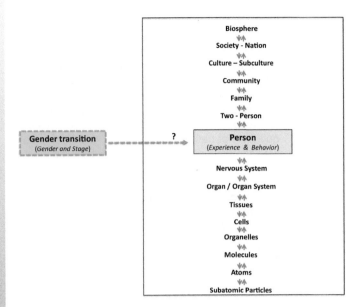

Fig. 2. It is unclear where gender transition fits into the original biopsychosocial model. (Reprinted with permission from the American Journal of Psychiatry, Volume 137, Issue 5, "The clinical application of the biopsychosocial model," p. 537 George L. Engel, (Copyright © 1980). American Psychiatric Association. All Rights Reserved.)

A Proposed Biopsychosocial Model for Transgender Health Care

George L Engel and Jon Romano proposed a systems model for medicine that focuses on the development of illness as arising from the complex interactions across and within biological, psychological, and social systems (**Fig. 1**).[79,80] Engel emphasized that the biomedical approach is flawed because the body is not the *only* contributor to illness or wellness.[80,81] Instead, an individual's own psychological (mood, personality, behavior, and so forth) and social (cultural, familial, socioeconomic, and so forth) domains *also* significantly impact underlying biological (genetic, biochemical, and so forth) factors to determine how illness and health are caused and treated.[79] Engel also emphasized the need for two-way dialogue between the patient and doctor to find the most effective treatments.[80]

What is perhaps *less* obvious from Engel and Romano's biopsychosocial model is that for people undergoing gender transition, the individual at the heart of the model can be different and changing at any given time (**Fig. 2**). It is useful for health care providers to consider how changes in sex hormones, body appearance, dress, personal pronouns, partner, family, and professional relations can occur during gender transition and that such changes affect health and illness. In essence, a provider can consider how each subdomain of Engel's biopsychosocial model is affected by the nature and stage of gender transition.

We note that the process of gender transition affects (and is affected by) both biological and social

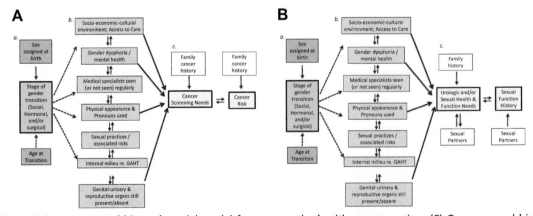

Fig. 3. (*A*) Our proposed biopsychosocial model for transgender health care screening. (*B*) Our proposed biopsychosocial model for transgender urologic and sexual health care.

Table 1
Best practices cancer screening protocol

Patients	Cancer Site	Population	Recommendation
Assigned Female at Birth	Colon	All patients over 50 y	Annual guaiac-based fecal occult blood test, or annual fecal immunochemical test, or multitarget stool DNA test every 3 y, or flexible sigmoidoscopy every 5 y, or double-contrast barium enema every 5 y, or colonoscopy every 10 y, or CT colonography every 5 y
	Lung	Patients who are current or former smokers ages 55–74 w/30 pack year history or quit smoking <15 y ago	Discuss annual screening with low-dose helical CT with physician
	Breast	Patients after bilateral mastectomy Patients before bilateral mastectomy or just underwent breast reduction	Currently no recommendations for this population Follow cis-female guidelines: • Age 40–44 y patients should have the option to undergo annual mammogram screening; • Age 45–54 y patients should undergo annual mammogram; • Patients age ≥55 y should transition to biennial mammograms as long as they are in good health
	Cervix	All patients age ≥21y that still have a cervix	Follow cis-female guidelines: • Age 21–29 y screening should be done every 3 y with Pap test • Age 30–65 y screening should be done every 5 y with both HPV DNA and Pap tests (preferred) or every 3 y with Pap test alone (acceptable)
	Ovary	All patients that still have ovaries	No recommended screening. Prophylactic oophorectomy not recommended
	Uterus	All patients that still have a uterus	Screening and prophylactic hysterectomy are not recommended Patients with a uterus should report any abnormal vaginal bleeding or discharge to a physician. Patients should undergo endometrial evaluation as a part of preoperative testing for genital gender affirmation surgery
	Prostate	N/A	—
	Anus	Men who have sex with men	No set guidelines, but this is an area of active research with the ANCHOR trial. At risk patients should discuss screening options (anal Pap smear and anoscopy) with their physician

(continued on next page)

Table 1
(*continued*)

Patients	Cancer Site	Population	Recommendation
Assigned Male at Birth	Colon	All patients over 50 y	Annual guaiac-based fecal occult blood test, or annual fecal immunochemical test, or multitarget stool DNA test every 3 y, or flexible sigmoidoscopy every 5 y, or double-contrast barium enema every 5 y, or colonoscopy every 10 y, or CT colonography every 5 y
	Lung	Patients who are current or former smokers ages 55–74 w/30 pack year history or quit smoking <15 y ago	Discuss annual screening with low-dose helical CT with physician
	Breast	Started GAHT	Follow cis-female guidelines: • Age 40–44 y patients should have the option to undergo annual mammogram screening; • Age 45–54 y patients should undergo annual mammogram; • Patients age ≥55 y should transition to biennial mammograms as long as they are in good health
	Prostate	All patients with a prostate	Follow cis-male guidelines (1 ng/mL should be the upper limit of normal in patients on GAH): • Age 40–49 y patients with family history or another high-risk feature should undergo annual PSA screening; • Age 50–74 y patients should undergo annual PSA check; • Age ≥75 y patients screening is an option if life expectancy >10 y
	Testicles	All patients with testicles	Annual physical examination for testicular masses
	Vagina	All patients with a neovagina	Annual postoperative physical examination (speculum and digital examination), cytology testing every 3 y starting at 21 y
	Anus	Patients age ≥21 y with multiple lifetime sexual partners	Annual anal Pap smear

HPV vaccination is recommended for all transgender individuals through age 26 y.

continua. For example, GAHT and surgery are a part of gender transition for many transgender or gender nonconforming people, as is a significant change in an individual's gender and social roles. A common theme in the WPATH SOC Guidelines is that a cornerstone of care for the transgender patient is to facilitate and adapt to positive change in mental health, social domains, and for some, physical/body-related domains.[5]

What is perhaps *less* obvious from the biopsychosocial model is that for people experiencing gender transition, certain subdomains of the biological and social continua change significantly and often over a relatively short period of time. It is useful for health care providers to consider how changes in sex hormones, body appearance, dress, personal pronouns, partner, family, and professional relations can occur during the transition process, and how such changes can affect health and illness.

We proposed a model for health care of the transgender and gender nonconforming individual that accounts for the complex interplay between the individual's gender transition, biological, and social systems (**Fig. 3**A, B). In the context of cancer screening, the model we proposed reminds us that cancer risk at any given time is influenced by the multiple levels of organization that Engel describes in the biopsychosocial model, in addition to, other factors specific to gender transition (see **Fig. 3**A).[82] For example, the age at which an individual commenced transition with use of GAHT, and the nature of their gender transition and what stages of transition they have completed, influence cancer risk (see **Fig. 3**A). Similarly, a transgender individual's urologic and sexual health/function needs will, at any given time, be defined by the state of their gender transition (see **Fig. 3**B).

When we consider transgender health from the perspective of the model shown in **Figs. 2** and **3**, three key points become clear. *First*, gender transition is highly individualized, and so must constitute different changes for different people. *Second*, at any given time that a patient interfaces with a health care provider, the patient may be in a different state of gender transition. *Third*, an individual's present state of gender transition independently influences (and is influenced by) each of the concentric levels of organization within the biological, psychological, and social continua that define the individual.

SUMMARY

Current evidence does not suggest that GAHT independently increases oncologic risks for transgender individuals. However, evidence is limited and further research into long-term effects of GAHT is needed. GAHT does not eliminate the malignancy potential of a patient's natal sex organs. Transgender individuals should undergo cancer screening for all present organs at risk for malignancy, regardless of transition status. Our proposed biopsychosocial model for transgender health care emphasizes that an individual's state of gender transition at any given time influences the concentric biological, psychological, and social hierarchical domains that constitute the individual. It is possible that a transgender patient's cancer risk can increase simply from failure to screen and detect malignancy. Established guidelines for cisgender individuals can reasonably be applied to transgender patients. Comprehensive cancer screening and prevention initiatives centered on relevant anatomy and high-risk behaviors specific for transgender men and women are needed (**Table 1**).

CLINICS CARE POINTS

- Summary of cancer screening recommendations for transmasculine and transfeminine patients

- All transgender and gender nonbinary patients should have an anatomic inventory conducted and appropriate cancer screening protocols should be practiced based on in situ anatomy.

- Although a theoretic cancer risk with GAHT may exist, no long-term studies demonstrate increased risks of cancer in patients on puberty blockers or long-term GAHT. Any discussion of theoretic malignancy risks should be balanced with discussions of the benefit of GAHT in treatment of gender dysphoria.

- Prospective trials are needed to formalize clear and consistent evidence-based cancer screening guidelines in the transgender population.

- What state of gender transition a patient exists in at any given time affects all biopsychosocial systems, as they relate to cancer and other urologic domains.

CONTRIBUTIONS

(I) Conception and design: All authors; (II) Administrative support: M.M. Garcia; (III) Provision of study materials or patients: J. Sterling; (IV) Collection and assembly of data: All authors; (V) Data analysis and interpretation: All authors; (VI) Manuscript writing: All authors; (VII) Final approval of manuscript: All authors.

FUNDING SOURCE

Grant from a research grant from Dr Richard Onofrio, MD to the Cedars-Sinai Medical Center Transgender Surgery and Health Program.

DECLARATION OF INTEREST

M.M. Garcia: (1) Co-Founder/Co-Inventor, Safe Medical Design, LLC; (2) Stockholder, MLM Sante, LLC; (3) P.I., NIH R01 1R01CA201709 to 0; (4) Honoraria for Education lectures, World Professional Association for Transgender Health.

REFERENCES

1. Zauber AG. The impact of screening on colorectal cancer mortality and incidence: has it really made a difference? Dig Dis Sci 2015;60(3):681–91.
2. de Koning HJ, Meza R, Plevritis SK, et al. Benefits and harms of computed tomography lung cancer screening strategies: a comparative modeling study for the U.S. Preventive Services Task Force. Ann Intern Med 2014;160(5):311–20.
3. Nelson HD, Fu R, Cantor A, et al. Effectiveness of Breast Cancer Screening: Systematic Review and Meta-analysis to Update the 2009 U.S. Preventive Services Task Force Recommendation. Ann Intern Med 2016;164(4):244–55.
4. Howlander N, Noone A, Krapcho M, et al. SEER cancer statsitics review. Bethesda, MD: National Cancer Institue; 2008.
5. Coleman E, Radix A, Bouman W, et al. Standards of care for the health of transgender and gender diverse people, version 8. International Journal of Transgender Health 2022;23(sup1):S1–259.
6. Saunders CL, Meads C, Abel GA, et al. Associations Between Sexual Orientation and Overall and Site-Specific Diagnosis of Cancer: Evidence From Two National Patient Surveys in England. J Clin Oncol 2017;35(32):3654–61.
7. Boehmer U, Miao X, Maxwell NI, et al. Sexual minority population density and incidence of lung, colorectal and female breast cancer in California. BMJ Open 2014;4(3):e004461.
8. Valanis BG, Bowen DJ, Bassford T, et al. Sexual orientation and health: comparisons in the women's health initiative sample. Arch Fam Med 2000;9(9):843–53.
9. Case P, Austin SB, Hunter DJ, et al. Sexual orientation, health risk factors, and physical functioning in the Nurses' Health Study II. J Womens Health (Larchmt) 2004;13(9):1033–47.
10. Cathcart-Rake EJ. Cancer in Sexual and Gender Minority Patients: Are We Addressing Their Needs? Curr Oncol Rep 2018;20(11):85.
11. CDC. CDC-Funded HIV testing: United States, Puerto Rico and the US Virgin Islands. 2015; Available at: http://www.cdc.gov/hiv/library/reports/index.html. Accessed April 22, 2023.
12. Clark H, Babu AS, Wiewel EW, et al. Diagnosed HIV Infection in Transgender Adults and Adolescents: Results from the National HIV Surveillance System, 2009-2014. AIDS Behav 2017;21(9):2774–83.
13. Becasen JS, Denard CL, Mullins MM, et al. Estimating the Prevalence of HIV and Sexual Behaviors Among the US Transgender Population: A Systematic Review and Meta-Analysis, 2006-2017. Am J Publ Health 2018;e1–8.
14. Tabaac AR, Sutter ME, Wall CSJ, et al. Gender Identity Disparities in Cancer Screening Behaviors. Am J Prev Med 2018;54(3):385–93.
15. Grant JMML, Mottet L, Tanis J, et al. National transgender discrimination survey report on health and health care.
16. Coleman E, Radix AE, Bouman WP, et al. Standards of Care for the Health of Transgender and Gender Diverse People. Int J Transgend Health 2022; 23(Suppl 1):S1–259. Version 8.
17. Arcelus J, Bouman WP, Van Den Noortgate W, et al. Systematic review and meta-analysis of prevalence studies in transsexualism. Eur Psychiatr 2015;30(6):807–15.
18. Zaliznyak M, Bresee C, Garcia MM. Age at first experience of gender dysphoria among transgender adults seeking gender-affirming surgery. JAMA Netw Open 2020;3(3):e201236.
19. Marshall SA, Allison MK, Stewart MK, et al. Highest Priority Health and Health Care Concerns of Transgender and Nonbinary Individuals in a Southern State. Transgend Health 2018;3(1):190–200.
20. Reisner SL, Poteat T, Keatley J, et al. Global health burden and needs of transgender populations: a review. Lancet 2016;388(10042):412–36.
21. Olson-Kennedy J, Okonta V, Clark LF, et al. Physiologic Response to Gender-Affirming Hormones Among Transgender Youth. J Adolesc Health 2018; 62(4):397–401.
22. McFarlane T, Zajac JD, Cheung AS. Gender-affirming hormone therapy and the risk of sex hormone-dependent tumours in transgender individuals-A systematic review. Clin Endocrinol 2018;89(6):700–11.
23. Nelson B. Troubling blind spots in understanding cancer risks among transgender patients: Bias, discrimination, and a lack of good data may be impeding cancer screening and risk assessments for the transgender population. In this article, the second of a 2-part series, we explore the remaining gaps in understanding and communicating the risks. Cancer Cytopathol 2019;127(8):487–8.
24. Jarin J. The Ob/Gyn and the transgender patient. Curr Opin Obstet Gynecol 2019;31(5):298–302.

25. Vermeulen MA, Slaets L, Cardoso F, et al. Pathological characterisation of male breast cancer: Results of the EORTC 10085/TBCRC/BIG/NABCG International Male Breast Cancer Program. Eur J Cancer 2017;82:219–27.

26. Chia K, O'Brien M, Brown M, et al. Targeting the androgen receptor in breast cancer. Curr Oncol Rep 2015;17(2):4.

27. de Blok CJM, Dreijerink KMA, den Heijer M. Cancer Risk in Transgender People. Endocrinol Metab Clin N Am 2019;48(2):441–52.

28. Gooren L, Morgentaler A. Prostate cancer incidence in orchidectomised male-to-female transsexual persons treated with oestrogens. Andrologia 2014; 46(10):1156–60.

29. Gooren LJ, van Trotsenburg MA, Giltay EJ, et al. Breast cancer development in transsexual subjects receiving cross-sex hormone treatment. J Sex Med 2013;10(12):3129–34.

30. Smith RA, Andrews KS, Brooks D, et al. Cancer screening in the United States, 2017: A review of current American Cancer Society guidelines and current issues in cancer screening. CA Cancer J Clin 2017;67(2):100–21.

31. Watanabe S, Teraishi F, Fujimoto S, et al. A Case of a Transwoman with Colorectal Cancer after Flap Vaginoplasty. J Plast Reconstr Aesthet Surg 2023;2(3): 98–101.

32. Newman PA, Roberts KJ, Masongsong E, et al. Anal Cancer Screening: Barriers and Facilitators Among Ethnically Diverse Gay, Bisexual, Transgender, and Other Men Who Have Sex With Men. J Gay Lesb Soc Serv 2008;20(4):328–53.

33. Kobayashi T, Sigel K, Gaisa M. Prevalence of Anal Dysplasia in Human Immunodeficiency Virus-Infected Transgender Women. Sex Transm Dis 2017;44(11): 714–6.

34. Ruanpeng D, Chariyalertsak S, Kaewpoowat Q, et al. Cytological Anal Squamous Intraepithelial Lesions Associated with Anal High-Risk Human Papillomavirus Infections among Men Who Have Sex with Men in Northern Thailand. PLoS One 2016;11(5):e0156280.

35. Thompson AB, Gillespie SE, Mosunjac MB, et al. Prevalence of Anal Squamous Intraepithelial Lesions in HIV-1-Infected Young Men Who Have Sex With Men and Transwomen. J Low Genit Tract Dis 2018;22(4):340–7.

36. Olsen CM, Green AC, Nagle CM, et al. Epithelial ovarian cancer: testing the 'androgens hypothesis. Endocr Relat Cancer 2008;15(4):1061–8.

37. Grynberg M, Fanchin R, Dubost G, et al. Histology of genital tract and breast tissue after long-term testosterone administration in a female-to-male transsexual population. Reprod Biomed Online 2010;20(4):553–8.

38. Brown GR. Breast Cancer in Transgender Veterans: A Ten-Case Series. LGBT Health 2015;2(1):77–80.

39. de Blok CJM, Wiepjes CM, Nota NM, et al. Breast cancer risk in transgender people receiving hormone treatment: nationwide cohort study in the Netherlands. BMJ 2019;365:l1652.

40. Nikolic DV, Djordjevic ML, Granic M, et al. Importance of revealing a rare case of breast cancer in a female to male transsexual after bilateral mastectomy. World J Surg Oncol 2012;10:280.

41. Kopetti C, Schaffer C, Zaman K, et al. Invasive Breast Cancer in a Trans Man After Bilateral Mastectomy: Case Report and Literature Review. Clin Breast Cancer 2021;21(3):e154–7.

42. Expert Panel on Breast I, Brown A, Lourenco AP, et al. ACR Appropriateness Criteria(R) Transgender Breast Cancer Screening. J Am Coll Radiol 2021; 18(11S):S502–15.

43. Salibian AA, Axelrod DM, Smith JA, et al. Oncologic Considerations for Safe Gender-Affirming Mastectomy: Preoperative Imaging, Pathologic Evaluation, Counseling, and Long-Term Screening. Plast Reconstr Surg 2021;147(2):213e–21e.

44. James S, Herman J, Rankin S, et al. The report of the 2015 US transgender survey. 2016.

45. Urban RR, Teng NN, Kapp DS. Gynecologic malignancies in female-to-male transgender patients: the need of original gender surveillance. Am J Obstet Gynecol 2011;204(5):e9–12.

46. Grimstad FW, Fowler KG, New EP, et al. Uterine pathology in transmasculine persons on testosterone: a retrospective multicenter case series. Am J Obstet Gynecol 2019;220(3):257.e1-7.

47. Peitzmeier SM, Khullar K, Reisner SL, et al. Pap test use is lower among female-to-male patients than non-transgender women. Am J Prev Med 2014; 47(6):808–12.

48. Porsch LM, Dayananda I, Dean G. An Exploratory Study of Transgender New Yorkers' Use of Sexual Health Services and Interest in Receiving Services at Planned Parenthood of New York City. Transgend Health 2016;1(1):231–7.

49. Gatos KC. A Literature Review of Cervical Cancer Screening in Transgender Men. Nurs Womens Health 2018;22(1):52–62.

50. Peitzmeier SM, Reisner SL, Harigopal P, et al. Female-to-male patients have high prevalence of unsatisfactory Paps compared to non-transgender females: implications for cervical cancer screening. J Gen Intern Med 2014;29(5):778–84.

51. Hembree WC, Cohen-Kettenis P, Delemarre-van de Waal HA, et al. Endocrine treatment of transsexual persons: an Endocrine Society clinical practice guideline. J Clin Endocrinol Metab 2009;94(9): 3132–54.

52. Wilson M, Berwick DM, DiGuiseppi C. The new edition of the Guide to Clinical Preventive Services. Pediatrics 1996;97(5):733–5.

53. Harris M, Kondel L, Dorsen C. Pelvic pain in transgender men taking testosterone: Assessing the risk of ovarian cancer. Nurs Pract 2017;42(7):1–5.

54. Joint R, Chen ZE, Cameron S. Breast and reproductive cancers in the transgender population: a systematic review. BJOG 2018;125(12):1505–12.

55. Blondeel K, Say L, Chou D, et al. Evidence and knowledge gaps on the disease burden in sexual and gender minorities: a review of systematic reviews. Int J Equity Health 2016;15(1):16.

56. Braun H, Nash R, Tangpricha V, et al. Cancer in Transgender People: Evidence and Methodological Considerations. Epidemiol Rev 2017;39(1):93–107.

57. Kvach EJ, Hyer JS, Carey JC, et al. Testicular Seminoma in a Transgender Woman: A Case Report. LGBT Health 2019;6(1):40–2.

58. Wolf-Gould CS, Wolf-Gould CH. A Transgender Woman with Testicular Cancer: A New Twist on an Old Problem. LGBT Health 2016;3(1):90–5.

59. Huggins C, Hodges CV. Studies on prostatic cancer: I. The effect of castration, of estrogen and of androgen injection on serum phosphatases in metastatic carcinoma of the prostate. 1941. J Urol 2002; 168(1):9–12.

60. Bosland MC. A perspective on the role of estrogen in hormone-induced prostate carcinogenesis. Cancer Lett 2013;334(1):28–33.

61. Hu WY, Shi GB, Lam HM, et al. Estrogen-initiated transformation of prostate epithelium derived from normal human prostate stem-progenitor cells. Endocrinology 2011;152(6):2150–63.

62. Rastrelli G, Corona G, Vignozzi L, et al. Serum PSA as a Predictor of Testosterone Deficiency. J Sex Med 2013;10(10):2518–28.

63. Nik-Ahd F, Jarjour A, Figueiredo J, et al. Prostate-Specific Antigen Screening in Transgender Patients. Eur Urol 2023;83(1):48–54.

64. Sterling J, Garcia MM. Cancer screening in the transgender population: a review of current guidelines, best practices, and a proposed care model. Transl Androl Urol 2020;9(6):2771–85.

65. Wittmann D, Mehta A, McCaughan E, et al. Guidelines for Sexual Health Care for Prostate Cancer Patients: Recommendations of an International Panel. J Sex Med 2022;19(11):1655–69.

66. Trum HW, Hoebeke P, Gooren LJ. Sex reassignment of transsexual people from a gynecologist's and urologist's perspective. Acta Obstet Gynecol Scand 2015;94(6):563–7.

67. Coleman E, Bockting W, Botzer M, et al. Standards of Care for the Health of Transsexual, Transgender, and Gender-Nonconforming People, Version 7. Int J Transgenderism 2012;13(4):165–232.

68. Deutsch MB, Radix A, Wesp L. Breast Cancer Screening, Management, and a Review of Case Study Literature in Transgender Populations. Semin Reprod Med 2017;35(5):434–41.

69. Colebunders B, T'Sjoen G, Weyers S, et al. Hormonal and surgical treatment in trans-women with BRCA1 mutations: a controversial topic. J Sex Med 2014;11(10):2496–9.

70. Fierz R, Ghisu GP, Fink D. Squamous Carcinoma of the Neovagina after Male-to-Female Reconstruction Surgery: A Case Report and Review of the Literature. Case Rep Obstet Gynecol 2019;2019:4820396.

71. Yamada K, Shida D, Kato T, et al. Adenocarcinoma arising in sigmoid colon neovagina 53 years after construction. World J Surg Oncol 2018;16(1):88.

72. Bogliolo S, Gaggero CR, Nadalini C, et al. Long-term risk of malignancy in the neovagina created using colon graft in vaginal agenesis - A case report. J Obstet Gynaecol 2015;35(5):543–4.

73. Grosse A, Grosse C, Lenggenhager D, et al. Cytology of the neovagina in transgender women and individuals with congenital or acquired absence of a natural vagina. Cytopathology 2017;28(3):184–91.

74. Brown B, Poteat T, Marg L, et al. Human Papillomavirus-Related Cancer Surveillance, Prevention, and Screening Among Transgender Men and Women: Neglected Populations at High Risk. LGBT Health 2017;4(5):315–9.

75. Frisch M, Biggar RJ, Goedert JJ. Human papillomavirus-associated cancers in patients with human immunodeficiency virus infection and acquired immunodeficiency syndrome. J Natl Cancer Inst 2000;92(18):1500–10.

76. Puechl AM, Russell K, Gray BA. Care and Cancer Screening of the Transgender Population. J Womens Health (Larchmt) 2019;28(6):761–8.

77. Unger CA. Care of the transgender patient: the role of the gynecologist. Am J Obstet Gynecol 2014; 210(1):16–26.

78. Compton ML, Taylor SS, Weeks AG, et al. Cytology and LGBT+ health: establishing inclusive cancer screening programs. J Am Soc Cytopathol 2022; 11(5):241–52.

79. Engel GL. The need for a new medical model: a challenge for biomedicine. Science 1977;196(4286): 129–36.

80. Engel GL. The clinical application of the biopsychosocial model. Am J Psychiatr 1980;137(5): 535–44.

81. Borrell-Carrio F, Suchman AL, Epstein RM. The biopsychosocial model 25 years later: principles, practice, and scientific inquiry. Ann Fam Med 2004;2(6): 576–82.

82. Lehman BJ, David DM, Gruber JA. Rethinking the biopsychosocial model of health: Understanding health as a dynamic system. Social and personality psychology compass 2017;11(8):e12328.

A Urologist's Guide to Caring for Transgender and Gender Diverse Patients

Fenizia Maffucci, MD[a], Jessica Clark, MD[a], Min Jun, DO[b],
Laura Douglass, MD[a],*

KEYWORDS

- Transgender health • Gender-affirming care • Gender-affirming surgery

KEY POINTS

- Urologists should understand the basic tenets of gender-affirming care and genital gender-affirming surgery.
- Feminizing genital procedures include orchiectomy and vaginoplasty. Masculinizing genital procedures include metoidioplasty, phalloplasty, and insertion of penile and testicular prostheses.
- Urologists can manage many surgical issues related to gender-affirming procedures. Urologists can also manage voiding dysfunction, recurrent urinary tract infections, fertility preservation, and urologic cancer screening for transgender and gender diverse patients.

INTRODUCTION

According to the World Professional Association for Transgender Health (WPATH), the term *transgender* describes people with gender identities or expressions that differ from the sex assigned at birth.[1] Recent studies estimate that 0.58% of adults (1.4 million people) in the United States of America currently identify as transgender.[2]

Those who identify as transgender may face discrimination across diverse sectors spanning housing, employment, education, criminal justice, and health care.[2,3] Historically, health care systems have not been inclusive of transgender patients. In a landmark survey of transgender individuals by the National Center for Transgender Equality and the National Gay and Lesbian Task Force, approximately 28% of respondents reported that they were subjected to gender-based harassment in medical settings.[3]

Urologists, as experts in the fields of genital and pelvic anatomy, sexual health and reproductive medicine, are uniquely poised to advance care for transgender individuals. Urologists routinely provide gender-affirming care—examples include managing testosterone deficiency with hormone replacement therapy and treatment of erectile dysfunction for cisgender men. Urologists have a responsibility to extend their expertise to be inclusive of transgender and gender diverse individuals.

While additional training is recommended to perform major genital gender-affirming procedures such as vaginoplasty or phalloplasty, this article will review the fundamentals necessary for the general urologist to appropriately manage basic surgical issues and common urologic conditions in transgender and gender diverse patients.

LANGUAGE AND TERMINOLOGY

An inclusive practice is built upon a foundation of appropriate terminology and language, as listed in **Table 1**. Language is constantly evolving, and some patients may use different terminology. Respecting the language patients use to describe

[a] Department of Urology, Lewis Katz School of Medicine at Temple University, 3401 North Broad Street, Philadelphia, PA 19140, USA; [b] Crane Center for Transgender Surgery, 575 Sir Francis Drake Boulevard, Suite 1, Greenbrae, CA 94904, USA
* Corresponding author.
E-mail address: Laura.Douglass@tuhs.temple.edu

Urol Clin N Am 50 (2023) 577–585
https://doi.org/10.1016/j.ucl.2023.06.020
0094-0143/23/© 2023 Elsevier Inc. All rights reserved.

Table 1
Essential terms and definitions[1,4–6]

Term	Definition
Sex	Refers to anatomical, physiologic, or genetic factors that define a person as female, male, or intersex independent of one's self-identity.
Sex assigned at birth	Refers to the sex given at birth, often based on the phenotype of the child's genitalia and/or the child's chromosomes.
Sexual orientation	Refers to a person's sexual, romantic and/or emotional attraction to people of certain genders or sexes on a spectrum. This can include lesbian, gay, bisexual, pansexual, or straight orientations. This is independent from a person's gender identity.
Gender	Refers to the social or behavioral norms that a culture associates typically with males or females. This can also refer to social or behavioral norms considered non-binary (not strictly male or female).
Gender identity	Refers to one's inner sense of self as being male, female, or non-binary on a spectrum. This may not be apparent to others. This can be fixed or fluid.
Gender expression	Refers to how a person presents themselves via behaviors, speech, clothing, or other characteristics that may be associated as feminine, masculine, or gender non-conforming.
Cisgender	Refers to a person whose gender identity aligns with the sex assigned at birth.
Transgender	Refers to a person whose gender identity differs from the sex assigned at birth.
Gender dysphoria	Refers to the distress related to incongruence between a person's gender identity and the sex assigned at birth. Not all transgender people experience gender dysphoria.
Gender-affirming care	Refers to a range of social, behavioral, and medical interventions that support and affirm a person's gender identity.
Gender-affirming surgery	Refers to surgical procedures that aim to better align a patient's physical characteristics with their gender identity.

their own experiences, identities or body parts is recommended.

Pronouns and Names

Using appropriate pronouns and names in reference to a person communicates understanding and respect.

Pronouns are words that refer to person(s) in the first, second, or third person. Gender is often implied. There are a variety of pronouns used in the transgender and gender diverse community including "he/him", "she/her" and "they/them".

The Electronic Medical Record (EMR) typically contains a patient's legal name from state-issued identification or from their insurance card, which may differ from the name the patient uses. This can lead to incorrect use of names and pronouns. Office intake forms that allow patients to self-identify name, pronouns, and gender identity are helpful.

When meeting a new patient, a provider should introduce themselves and the pronouns they use, and then ask patients their names and pronouns. If an error is made, a simple apology and correction is recommended. If one notices others using incorrect language to reference a patient, a correction should be offered.

GENDER-AFFIRMING CARE

Gender-affirming care refers to a range of social, behavioral, and medical interventions that support and affirm the expression of a person's gender identity. Many transgender individuals will pursue various medical interventions–such as hormone therapy and gender-affirming surgery–to better align their physical body with their gender identity. Transgender patients are not homogenous, and individual goals and needs should guide their care. Understanding the basic tenets of gender-affirming care can help urologists provide competent care related to surgical or general urologic issues.

Hormone Therapy

Hormone therapy is a tool to promote the development of desired secondary sex characteristics while reducing undesired secondary sex characteristics. When provided under medical supervision by an experienced provider, hormone therapy in adults is safe.[7–9] Expected effects vary across individuals and are typically seen over several years of use.[10,11] Some effects are contingent on continued usage, while others are irreversible.

Feminizing hormone therapy typically includes estrogen and an anti-androgen.[1] Some patients may elect to undergo an orchiectomy, either alone or as part of vaginoplasty. Expected changes include breast growth to variable degrees, decreased testicular size, decreased libido, and increased ratio of subcutaneous body fat to muscle mass.[10,12,13]

Estrogen use is associated with an increased risk of venous thromboembolism (VTE).[14,15] One meta-analysis found the incidence of VTE in transgender women using estrogen to be 2.3 events per 1000 person years.[16] This risk may be compounded by smoking, obesity, or personal or family history of thrombosis.[15,16] To decrease the chances of developing VTE, modifiable risk factors should be optimized and less thrombogenic formulations of estrogen should be considered.[15–17]

Currently, there is no evidence demonstrating increased VTE in patients who continue gender-affirming estrogen use perioperatively compared to those who hold their estrogen.[15,18–20] Continuing estrogen through surgery and recovery has the potential benefits of decreasing dysphoria and anxiety. Appropriate VTE prophylaxis is recommended including sequential compression devices, heparin or enoxaparin, and early ambulation.

Masculinizing hormone therapy consists of testosterone which results in variable clitoral enlargement, increased libido, a deepened voice, growth of body and facial hair, cessation of menses, atrophy of breast tissue and decreased mass of body fat.[9,13,21,22] Testosterone use can be associated with polycythemia and hypertension.[23] Patients must be closely monitored for changes to their blood pressure, lipid panels, and hematocrit.[23]

Surgery

Gender-affirming surgery (GAS) refers to procedures that better align a patient's physical characteristics with their gender identity. GAS includes craniofacial procedures, chest procedures, and genital procedures.

The WPATH releases Standards of Care (SOC), which are evidence-based guidelines with proposed criteria for patients seeking GAS. The updated SOC Version 8 recommends individuals who fulfill criteria for GAS to obtain one letter of assessment from a healthcare professional with competency in the assessment of transgender and gender diverse people.[1] The guidelines also suggest that a patient seeking gonadectomy should be stable on their hormone regimen for a minimum of 6 months prior to surgery unless hormones are not desired or are contraindicated.[1]

Feminizing Genital Gender-Affirming Surgery: Orchiectomy and Vaginoplasty

Orchiectomy

Some trans-feminine or non-binary individuals will elect to undergo bilateral orchiectomy. Removal of the gonads often allows patients to stop taking antiandrogens and to decrease their dose of estrogen.[24] Patients may choose to undergo orchiectomy as their only form of gender-affirming genital surgery, orchiectomy prior to future vaginoplasty, or orchiectomy at the time of vaginoplasty.

Orchiectomy is an opportunity for general urologists to provide GAS, especially in locations without major GAS centers. Before performing gender-affirming orchiectomy, urologists should inquire about a patient's desire for fertility preservation (see the section on Fertility Preservation). The authors recommend performing orchiectomy through a single midline high scrotal or penoscrotal incision to minimize scarring of scrotal skin, which may be used as a skin graft in future vaginoplasty. Ligation of the spermatic cord should be performed close to the external inguinal ring to prevent a palpable cord stump. Efforts to preserve surrounding tissues is recommended, as it will help provide fullness to the labia majora for future vaginoplasty.[25]

Vaginoplasty

Vaginoplasty refers to the construction of an external vulva and a vaginal canal. If no vaginal canal is to be created, then the procedure is referred to as a vulvoplasty, or "zero depth" or "shallow depth" vaginoplasty.

Given its complexity and risk of complications, vaginoplasty should be performed by surgeons with formal training in GAS. A recent systematic review and meta-analysis by Manrique and colleagues[26] reported the following rates of post-vaginoplasty complications: 10% stenosis or stricture, 3% prolapse, 2% tissue necrosis, and 1% rectovaginal fistula. Wound complications are common–granulation tissue externally and within the vaginal canal can be addressed with silver nitrate, debridement, or topical steroids.[27] Because the vaginal canal is created between the urinary tract and rectum, related complications may be encountered. If foley catheter placement is required in a patient post-vaginoplasty, the pink mucosa of the urethral plate can help identify the urethral meatus which is located just above the vaginal introitus.

When seeing patients who underwent vaginoplasty, urologists should be aware that a combination of penile skin and scrotal skin grafts are used to line the vaginal canal. Additional skin grafts from the lower abdomen, groin, or thigh may be utilized. Robotic peritoneal flap vaginoplasty is an increasingly popular technique in which flaps of peritoneum are created and attached to the inverted penile skin tube to create the vaginal canal.[28] Efforts should be made to preserve the blood supply to flaps and grafts if operating in these areas.

Masculinizing Genital Procedures: Metoidioplasty, Phalloplasty

There are many masculinizing genital procedures including hysterectomy, salpingo-oophorectomy, vaginectomy, colpocleisis, metoidioplasty, phalloplasty, scrotoplasty, testicular implants and penile implants. The selection of procedures is highly dependent on achieving a patient's specific goals, which can include good cosmetic appearance, standing with urination, achieving erections and/or intromission while maintaining sensation and the ability to orgasm.[29,30]

Herein, we will focus on urologic aspects of metoidioplasty, phalloplasty, testicular implants and penile implants.

Metoidioplasty

Metoidioplasty is the creation of a neophallus using the hormonally enlarged clitoris, typically in 1 or 2 stages. The length of the neophallus is dependent on the patient's existing anatomy and surgical technique. Neophallus length has been reported to range from 4–10 cm (1.6–3.9 inches), and typically does not allow for penetrative intercourse.[31] The dorsal neurovascular bundle is preserved, and erogenous sensation and ability to orgasm are maintained.[31] For patients who desire standing to void, urethral lengthening is performed utilizing techniques similar to hypospadias repair.[31–33] Scrotoplasty can also be performed using various techniques to mobilize labia majora tissues, with or without testicular implants.

Metoidioplasty avoids donor site morbidity and scarring while allowing shorter recovery and less stages compared to phalloplasty.[34] Patients can also undergo phalloplasty in the future with good outcomes.[35,36]

Complications of metoidioplasty include urethral fistula or strictures. One major high-volume center reported outcomes of 813 patients who underwent one-stage metoidioplasty over a 14-year period and found that urethral fistula and stricture occurred in 8.85% and 1.70% of cases, respectively.[35] If there is concern for urinary retention, urinary fistula or urethral stricture in a patient with urethral lengthening, placement of a suprapubic catheter is likely safer and preferred in most cases. If a urethral catheter is required, the authors would consider using a flexible ureteroscope to gain access into the bladder or one attempt at gentle blind passage of a 14Fr silicone catheter.

Phalloplasty

Phalloplasty involves creation of a neophallus, most commonly with a radial forearm free flap (RFFF) or an anterolateral thigh (ALT) flap.[37]

Neophallus length is longer following phalloplasty compared to metoidioplasty and can accommodate penile prosthesis implantation and penetrative intercourse.[38,39] A recent meta-analysis reported a mean length of approximately 13 cm (5.1 inches) following phalloplasty.[40] However, phalloplasty is a complex surgical undertaking that involves multiple stages with higher rates of complications compared to metoidioplasty.[40]

Many patients will pursue urethral lengthening in one or multiple stages to stand to void. Urethral segments include the pars fixa (non-mobile perineal portion of the neourethra which connects the native urethra to the pars pendulans) and the pars pendulans (portion of the neourethra within the neophallus).[34,41] Urethral anastomoses between the native urethra to the pars fixa, and the pars fixa to the pars pendulans are vascular watershed areas vulnerable to both fistula and stricture.[42,43] The urethral meatus is also prone to stricture. To minimize these complications, tensionless closure and preservation of a robust blood supply are prioritized.[42–44]

A recent meta-analysis reported an approximately 76.5% overall complication rate following phalloplasty.[40] Urethral complications are common, including a fistula rate of 34% and a stricture rate of 25%.[40] If there is concern for urethral complications following urethral lengthening, a suprapubic tube should be favored over a urethral catheter as previously discussed.[44,45]

Small fistulas may spontaneously resolve with urinary diversion with a suprapubic catheter.[34] Those that do not heal will require surgical repair by reconstructive urologists. Urethral strictures will not be intervened on for at least 3 months following phalloplasty to allow time for blood supply to develop.[34,42]

Additionally, patients who have undergone urethral lengthening may experience pooling of urine in the transition point from the compliant native urethra and the poorly compliant neourethra resulting in post void dribbling. Manual "milking" of the neourethra at the base of the reconstructed scrotum may help.[30] Leakage of urine after voiding may also indicate pooling of urine in a persistent vaginal remnant.[46]

Testicular and Penile Prosthesis

Patients may elect for testicular prostheses while undergoing scrotoplasty. Testicular implants carry a relatively small risk of complications–a high volume center reported 4% risk of displacement and 1% risk of rejection.[31]

There are significant anatomical differences between a neophallus and a natal penis which make penile prosthesis implantation challenging. There is a lack of divergent penile crura which makes it difficult to anchor the proximal end of a penile implant.[38] Neophalluses also lack tunica albuginea which provide protection against distal protrusion and erosion.[38] Dilation must occur with great care to avoid perforation. An infrapubic approach is typically utilized to avoid the vascular pedicle flap.[38,39]

A recent review reported that the rate of inflatable penile prosthetic revision or replacement in transgender men is approximately 23 – 70%.[38] The long-term reliability and longevity of penile prostheses in transgender individuals has not been well studied.

Complications of penile prosthesis are handled similarly in the transgender and cisgender population. Mild skin infections can be treated with a trial of antibiotics and significant infections require removal of all hardware. Erosion requires revision and re-positioning of the prosthesis or complete removal.[47,48] When performing explantation of a penile prosthesis in a patient who underwent phalloplasty, the urologist must consider the location of the vascular pedicle and avoid it. Communication with the original surgeon is recommended if surgery must be performed emergently.

GENERAL UROLOGIC CARE

Urologists should be prepared to care for common urologic issues in transgender and gender diverse patients in a variety of practice settings.

History

Gather a detailed medical history including a history of gender-affirming care. Inquire about duration of hormone therapy and if the patient underwent any genital GAS. The authors recommend taking note of a patient's "organ inventory," and clarify which organs they have in place and which ones have been removed (**Table 2**).[10] Understanding a patient's anatomy will help guide your physical examination and recommendations.

Physical Examination

Pelvic and genital examinations may trigger dysphoria and can be a source of trauma for transgender patients. When examining a transgender individual, one should provide a safe and inclusive environment. When possible, use gender neutral terms to describe anatomy. For example, rather than using the word "penis" or "vulva," consider using the term "external genitalia." Rather than "testicles" or "ovaries," use the term "gonads."[10,49] It is always best to ask what terms patients prefer to use in reference to their bodies.

Physical examinations should be focused. Discuss the rationale and steps of the examination, and obtain consent. If needed, a support person and/or an oral benzodiazepine for anxiety may be helpful. The authors recommend having a chaperone present.

Urinary/Voiding Symptoms

Transgender patients can experience lower urinary symptoms for a variety of reasons.

Trans-feminine patients (which can include transgender women and feminine-presenting nonbinary individuals) often take spironolactone as an antiandrogen and may develop urinary frequency due to its diuretic effects.[50] Discussion with their hormone provider regarding alternative antiandrogens may be helpful, as well as considering orchiectomy. Patients may have smaller prostate glands because of hormone therapy and are less likely to have prostatic obstruction as the etiology of lower urinary symptoms.[51] Consider voiding dysfunction and pelvic floor

Table 2 Example of an "organ inventory"[10]	
Organs	**Alternative Gender-Neutral Terms**
Breast	Chest, top, upper body
Vulva	External genitals
Vagina	Internal genitals
Cervix	Internal reproductive organs
Uterus	Internal reproductive organs
Ovaries	Internal gonads
Testicles	External gonads
Prostate	Internal reproductive organs
Penis	External genitals, erectile tissue

dysfunction as possible causes. Urodynamics and cystoscopy may be helpful to guide diagnosis and management.

After vaginoplasty, patients may experience post-operative acute urinary retention requiring temporary catheterization. Most cases of post-operative retention spontaneously resolve. Urethral stenosis and urinary stream issues can occur and may require additional procedures. Patients may develop new urinary symptoms such as overactive bladder and urinary incontinence after vaginoplasty and can be managed accordingly.[52] Patients may benefit from pelvic floor physical therapy.[53,54]

Trans-masculine patients (which can include transgender men and masculine-presenting nonbinary individuals) may present with urinary symptoms related to testosterone therapy and resultant atrophy of genital tissues, similar to the effects seen in the post-menopausal vaginal epithelium of cisgender women. These effects can be mitigated using topical estrogen, which has minimal systemic absorption.[10,55] Some patients may not be willing to insert estrogen into their genital region due to dysphoria.

After masculinizing genital gender-affirming surgery, urethral complications are common and may present with a wide range of urinary symptoms. Imaging with a retrograde urethrogram or voiding cystourethrogram may be helpful to delineate anatomy and assess for stricture or fistula. Urodynamics and flexible cystoscopy performed with a ureteroscope or pediatric cystoscope may also be useful.[30]

Recurrent Urinary Tract Infection

Trans-feminine patients who undergo vaginoplasty have several risk factors for urinary tract infections (UTI), including a shortened urethra which is anatomically closer to the anus than in cisgender women. Patients who undergo vaginoplasty also have different vaginal pH and flora than cisgender women, which may predispose them to UTIs.[55,56] Additionally, consider prostatitis in patients with recurrent UTIs who have a prostate.[52]

Transmasculine individuals who are using hormones may be at increased risk of UTI due to atrophy of genital tissues and can be managed with topical estrogen as discussed previously. In those patients who previously underwent masculinizing genital surgery, urethral complications should also be considered as the underlying cause of recurrent UTI.

Fertility Preservation

All patients should be counseled on fertility preservation before starting hormones and undergoing gonadectomy.[1]

Semen parameters may be impacted by estrogen use in transgender women, although evidence is limited.[57,58] Consider obtaining a baseline semen analysis, and if there is no viable sperm, recommend cessation of estrogen for at least 3 months before retrieving sperm for banking.[57] Of note, this may delay GAS and estrogen cessation may increase dysphoria.

Transgender men will see Gynecology providers for fertility preservation which can include oocyte or embryo freezing.[1] Return of normal ovarian function after cessation of testosterone can vary and is dependent on the patient's age and length of testosterone therapy.[46]

Prostate Cancer Screening

The risk of prostate cancer in transgender women is theorized to be lower than cisgender men due to effects of estrogen and androgen deprivation.[59,60] However, there are documented cases of prostate cancer in transgender women.[61] The development of prostate cancer in the setting of androgen deprivation suggests high risk disease and potentially castrate-resistant prostate cancer.[62]

Currently, there is no consensus from major urologic societies regarding prostate screening antigen (PSA) screening in transgender women. PSA levels are affected by feminizing hormone therapy, and a "normal" baseline has yet to be established. Some studies quote that PSA of ≥ 1 ng/mL in transgender women who are on hormonal therapy and/or underwent bilateral orchiectomy should prompt further investigation for prostate cancer.[51,63,64]

Digital rectal examination (DRE) may not be reliable in transgender women if they have undergone vaginoplasty.[51,65] In these individuals, a digital vaginal examination of the prostate can be considered.[51,63]

Modality of prostate biopsy should be selected based on a patient's individual anatomy, including presence or depth or a vaginal canal. Transrectal, transvaginal or transperineal prostate biopsy may be considered.[51,63]

If a patient is diagnosed with prostate cancer, an in-depth discussion should take place regarding oncologic treatment options in the setting of prior history of or desire for future genital GAS. Vulvoplasty after prostatectomy or radiation may be safer than vaginoplasty due to potential higher risk of rectal injury during vaginal canal dissection.[51] Radiation therapy may be the safest treatment option after vaginoplasty.

Additional research is needed to establish guidelines for prostate cancer screening and management in the transgender population.

SUMMARY

Transgender and gender diverse individuals are seeking gender-affirming care at higher rates.[66] While access to care is increasing in the United States, there are relatively few specialized centers offering gender-affirming surgery, requiring many patients to travel.[67] Patients may seek care from local urologists as they return home in addition to establishing general urologic care. With increased understanding of the urologic needs of transgender and gender diverse patients, the general urologist is uniquely equipped to deliver competent and affirming care.

CLINICS CARE POINTS

- Fertility preservation is important to consider prior to undergoing gender-affirming care with hormones and surgery.
- Transgender and gender diverse individuals can elect to undergo a variety of genital gender-affirming surgery (GAS).
- Common complications of masculinizing genital GAS include urethral stricture and fistula formation. Suprapubic tube is preferred to manage these complications.
- Special considerations must be taken when placing a penile prosthesis in a transgender patient due to the differences in the anatomy of the neophallus.
- There is no clear consensus for prostate cancer screening and diagnosis for transgender women.

DISCLOSURE

There are no financial or commercial conflicts of interest to disclose.

REFERENCES

1. Coleman E, Radix AE, Bouman WP, et al. Standards of care for the health of transgender and gender diverse people, version 8. Int J Transgend Health 2022;23(S1). https://doi.org/10.1080/26895269.2022.2100644.
2. Flores AR, Herman JL, Gates GJ, et al. How many adults identify as transgender in the United States? Los Angeles, CA: The Williams Institute; 2016. Authors provide a contemporary estimate of the prevalence of transgender individuals in the US. Published online 2017.
3. Grant JM, Mottet L, Tanis J, et al. Injustice at every turn: a report of the national transgender discrimination survey, Washington National Center for Transgender Equality and National Gay and Lesbian Task Force, 25, 2011: 32-86, 106-123, 158-172.
4. Gonzalez G, Anger J. Creating an Inclusive Urology Practice. Curr Bladder Dysfunct Rep 2023. https://doi.org/10.1007/s11884-023-00694-7.
5. Mcnamara MC, Ng H. Best practices in LGBT care: a guide for primary care physicians. Cleve Clin J Med 2016;83(7). https://doi.org/10.3949/ccjm.83a.15148.
6. American Psychiatric Association, Diagnostic and statistical manual of mental disorders, Washington, DC, 2022, DSM-5-TR.
7. Tangpricha V, den Heijer M. Oestrogen and anti-androgen therapy for transgender women. Lancet Diabetes Endocrinol 2017;5(4). https://doi.org/10.1016/S2213-8587(16)30319-9.
8. Safer JD, Tangpricha V. Care of the transgender patient. Ann Intern Med 2019;171(1). https://doi.org/10.7326/AITC201907020.
9. Hembree WC, Cohen-Kettenis PT, Gooren L, et al. Endocrine treatment of gender-dysphoric/gender-incongruent persons: an endocrine society clinical practice guideline. J Clin Endocrinol Metab 2017;102(11). https://doi.org/10.1210/jc.2017-01658.
10. Deutsch M. Guidelines for the Primary and Gender-Affirming Care of Transgender and Gender Nonbinary People. UCSF Gender Affirming Health Program, Department of Family and Community Medicine, University of California San Francisco. Published June 17, 2016. Available at: https://transcare.ucsf.edu/guidelines. Accessed April 12, 2023.
11. van Dijk D, Dekker MJHJ, Conemans EB, et al. Explorative prospective evaluation of short-term subjective effects of hormonal treatment in trans people—results from the european network for the investigation of gender incongruence. J Sex Med 2019;16(8). https://doi.org/10.1016/j.jsxm.2019.05.009.
12. Coxon J, Seal L. Hormone management of trans women. Trends in Urology & Men's Health 2018;9(6). https://doi.org/10.1002/tre.663.
13. De Blok CJM, Dijkman BAM, Wiepjes CM, et al. Sustained breast development and breast anthropometric changes in 3 years of gender-affirming hormone treatment. J Clin Endocrinol Metab 2021;106(2). https://doi.org/10.1210/clinem/dgaa841.
14. Gomes MPV, Deitcher SR. Risk of venous thromboembolic disease associated with hormonal contraceptives and hormone replacement therapy: a clinical review. Arch Intern Med 2004;164(18). https://doi.org/10.1001/archinte.164.18.1965.
15. Zucker R, Reisman T, Safer JD. Minimizing venous thromboembolism in feminizing hormone therapy: applying lessons from cisgender women and previous data. Endocr Pract 2021;27(6). https://doi.org/10.1016/j.eprac.2021.03.010.

16. Khan J, Schmidt RL, Spittal MJ, et al. Venous thrombotic risk in transgender women undergoing estrogen therapy: a systematic review and metaanalysis. Clin Chem 2019;65(1). https://doi.org/10.1373/clinchem.2018.288316.

17. Nota NM, Wiepjes CM, De Blok CJM, et al. Occurrence of acute cardiovascular events in transgender individuals receiving hormone therapy: results from a large cohort study. Circulation 2019;139(11). https://doi.org/10.1161/CIRCULATIONAHA.118.038584.

18. Kozato A, Conner Fox GW, Yong PC, et al. No venous thromboembolism increase among transgender female patients remaining on estrogen for gender-affirming surgery. J Clin Endocrinol Metab 2021;106(4). https://doi.org/10.1210/clinem/dgaa966.

19. Gaither TW, Awad MA, Osterberg EC, et al. Postoperative complications following primary penile inversion vaginoplasty among 330 male-to-female transgender patients. J Urol 2018;199(3). https://doi.org/10.1016/j.juro.2017.10.013.

20. Prince JCJ, Safer JD. Endocrine treatment of transgender individuals: current guidelines and strategies. Expert Rev Endocrinol Metab 2020;15(6). https://doi.org/10.1080/17446651.2020.1825075.

21. Kuper LE, Mathews S, Lau M. Baseline mental health and psychosocial functioning of transgender adolescents seeking gender-affirming hormone therapy. J Dev Behav Pediatr 2019;40(8). https://doi.org/10.1097/DBP.0000000000000697.

22. Taliaferro LA, McMorris BJ, Rider GN, et al. Risk and protective factors for self-harm in a population-based sample of transgender youth. Arch Suicide Res 2019,23(2). https://doi.org/10.1080/13811118.2018.1430639.

23. Banks K, Kyinn M, Leemaqz SY, et al. Blood pressure effects of gender-affirming hormone therapy in transgender and gender-diverse adults. Hypertension 2021. https://doi.org/10.1161/HYPERTENSIONAHA.120.16839.

24. Hehemann MC, Walsh TJ. Orchiectomy as bridge or alternative to vaginoplasty. Urol Clin 2019;46(4). https://doi.org/10.1016/j.ucl.2019.07.005.

25. van der Sluis WB, Steensma TD, Bouman MB. Orchiectomy in transgender individuals: a motivation analysis and report of surgical outcomes. Int J Transgend Health 2020;21(2). https://doi.org/10.1080/26895269.2020.1749921.

26. Manrique OJ, Adabi K, Martinez-Jorge J, et al. Complications and patient-reported outcomes in male-to-female vaginoplasty-where we are today: a systematic review and meta-analysis. Ann Plast Surg 2018;80(6). https://doi.org/10.1097/SAP.0000000000001393.

27. Hirotsu K, Kannan S, Brian Jiang SI. Treatment of hypertrophic granulation tissue. Dermatol Surg 2019;45(12). https://doi.org/10.1097/dss.0000000000002059.

28. Jacoby A, Maliha S, Granieri MA, et al. Robotic Davydov Peritoneal Flap Vaginoplasty For Augmentation Of Vaginal Depth In Feminizing Vaginoplasty. J Urol 2019;201(6). https://doi.org/10.1097/JU.0000000000000107.

29. Ganor O, Taghinia AH, Diamond DA, et al. Piloting a genital affirmation surgical priorities scale for trans masculine patients. Transgend Health 2019;4(1). https://doi.org/10.1089/trgh.2019.0038.

30. Schechter LS. *Gender confirmation surgery: principles and techniques for an emerging field*. Cham: Springer; 2020. p. 161–9. https://doi.org/10.1007/978-3-030-29093-1.

31. Djordjevic ML, Stojanovic B, Bizic M. Metoidioplasty: techniques and outcomes. Transl Androl Urol 2019;8(3). https://doi.org/10.21037/tau.2019.06.12.

32. Meltzer TR, Esmonde NO. Metoidioplasty using labial advancement flaps for urethroplasty. Plast Aesthet Res 2020;7. https://doi.org/10.20517/2347-9264.2020.122.

33. Vukadinovic V, Stojanovic B, Majstorovic M, et al. The role of clitoral anatomy in female to male sex reassignment surgery. Sci World J 2014;2014. https://doi.org/10.1155/2014/437378.

34. Jun MS, Crane CN, Santucci RA. What urologists need to know about female-to-male genital confirmation surgery (phalloplasty and metoidioplasty): Techniques, complications, and how to deal with them. Minerva Urol Nefrol 2020;72(1). https://doi.org/10.23736/S0393-2249.19.03611-7.

35. Bordas N, Stojanovic B, Bizic M, et al. Metoidioplasty: surgical options and outcomes in 813 cases. Front Endocrinol 2021;12. https://doi.org/10.3389/fendo.2021.760284.

36. Al-Tamimi M, Pigot GL, van der Sluis WB, et al. The Surgical techniques and outcomes of secondary phalloplasty after metoidioplasty in transgender men: an international, multi-center case series. J Sex Med 2019;16(11). https://doi.org/10.1016/j.jsxm.2019.07.027.

37. Boczar D, Huayllani MT, Saleem HY, et al. Surgical techniques of phalloplasty in transgender patients: a systematic review. Ann Transl Med 2021;9(7). https://doi.org/10.21037/atm-20-3527.

38. Kang A, Aizen JM, Cohen AJ, et al. Techniques and considerations of prosthetic surgery after phalloplasty in the transgender male. Transl Androl Urol 2019;8(3). https://doi.org/10.21037/tau.2019.06.02.

39. Purohit RS, Kent M, Djordjevic ML. Penile prosthesis in transgender men after phalloplasty. Indian J Plast Surg 2022;55(2):168–73. https://doi.org/10.1055/s-0041-1740523.

40. Wang AMQ, Tsang V, Mankowski P, et al. Outcomes following gender affirming phalloplasty: a systematic review and meta-analysis. Sex Med Rev 2022;10(4). https://doi.org/10.1016/j.sxmr.2022.03.002.

41. Zisman A, Baiocco JA, Purohit RS. Management of urethral strictures after masculinizing genital surgery in transgender men. Plast Aesthet Res 2022;9(9). https://doi.org/10.20517/2347-9264.2021.113.

42. Jun MS, Santucci RA. Urethral stricture after phalloplasty. Transl Androl Urol 2019;8(3). https://doi.org/10.21037/tau.2019.05.08.

43. Heston AL, Esmonde NO, Dugi DD, et al. Phalloplasty: techniques and outcomes. Transl Androl Urol 2019;8(3):254–65. https://doi.org/10.21037/tau.2019.05.05.

44. Chen ML, Reyblat P, Poh MM, et al. Overview of surgical techniques in gender-affirming genital surgery. Transl Androl Urol 2019;8(3). https://doi.org/10.21037/tau.2019.06.19.

45. Nikolavsky D, Yamaguchi Y, Levine JP, et al. Urologic sequelae following phalloplasty in transgendered patients. Urol Clin 2017;44(1). https://doi.org/10.1016/j.ucl.2016.08.006.

46. Anderson K, Krakowsky Y, Potter E, et al. Adult transgender care: a review for urologists. Canadian Urological Association Journal 2021;15(10). https://doi.org/10.5489/cuaj.6949.

47. Briles BL, Middleton RY, Celtik KE, et al. Penile prosthesis placement by a dedicated transgender surgery unit: a retrospective analysis of complications. J Sex Med 2022;19(4). https://doi.org/10.1016/j.jsxm.2022.01.518.

48. van der Sluis WB, Pigot GLS, Al-Tamimi M, et al. A retrospective cohort study on surgical outcomes of penile prosthesis implantation surgery in transgender men after phalloplasty. Urology 2019;132. https://doi.org/10.1016/j.urology.2019.06.010.

49. ACON. Trans-Affirming Clinical Language. TransHub. Published April 13, 2023. Available at: https://static1.squarespace.com/static/5d8c2136980d9708b9ba5cd3/t/5fc9a8282f5dbb44b77798d1/1607051305514/Trans+Affirming+Clinical+Language+Guide_Final.pdf. Accessed April 12, 2023.

50. Wang Y, Lipner SR. Retrospective analysis of adverse events with spironolactone in females reported to the United States Food and Drug Administration. Int J Womens Dermatol 2020;6(4). https://doi.org/10.1016/j.ijwd.2020.05.002.

51. Bertoncelli Tanaka M, Sahota K, Burn J, et al. Prostate cancer in transgender women: what does a urologist need to know? BJU Int 2022;129(1). https://doi.org/10.1111/bju.15521.

52. Kreines FM, Hughes-Hogan L, Cifuentes M. Lower urinary tract symptoms after vaginoplasty: a review. Curr Bladder Dysfunct Rep 2022;17(2). https://doi.org/10.1007/s11884-022-00648-5.

53. Jiang DD, Gallagher S, Burchill L, et al. Implementation of a pelvic floor physical therapy program for transgender women undergoing gender-affirming vaginoplasty. Obstet Gynecol 2019;133. https://doi.org/10.1097/AOG.0000000000003236.

54. Manrique OJ, Adabi K, Huang TCT, et al. Assessment of pelvic floor anatomy for male-to-female vaginoplasty and the role of physical therapy on functional and patient-reported outcomes. Ann Plast Surg 2019;82(6). https://doi.org/10.1097/SAP.0000000000001680.

55. Krakowsky Y, Potter E, Hallarn J, et al. The effect of gender-affirming medical care on the vaginal and neovaginal microbiomes of transgender and gender-diverse people. Front Cell Infect Microbiol 2022;11. https://doi.org/10.3389/fcimb.2021.769950.

56. Birse KD, Kratzer K, Zuend CF, et al. The neovaginal microbiome of transgender women post-gender reassignment surgery. Microbiome 2020;8(1). https://doi.org/10.1186/s40168-020-00804-1.

57. Sterling J, Garcia MM. Fertility preservation options for transgender individuals. Transl Androl Urol 2020;9. https://doi.org/10.21037/tau.2019.09.28.

58. Adeleye AJ, Reid G, Kao CN, et al. Semen parameters among transgender women with a history of hormonal treatment. Urology 2019;124. https://doi.org/10.1016/j.urology.2018.10.005.

59. Jackson SS, Nambiar KZ, O'Callaghan S, et al. Understanding the role of sex hormones in cancer for the transgender community. Trends Cancer 2022;8(4). https://doi.org/10.1016/j.trecan.2022.01.005.

60. de Nie I, de Blok CJM, van der Sluis TM, et al. Prostate cancer incidence under androgen deprivation: nationwide cohort study in trans women receiving hormone treatment. J Clin Endocrinol Metab 2020;105(9). https://doi.org/10.1210/clinem/dgaa412.

61. Deebel NA, Morin JP, Autorino R, et al. Prostate cancer in transgender women: incidence, etiopathogenesis, and management challenges. Urology 2017;110. https://doi.org/10.1016/j.urology.2017.08.032.

62. Gaglani S, Purohit RS, Tewari AK, et al. Embryologic and hormonal contributors to prostate cancer in transgender women. Am J Clin Exp Urol 2022;10(2):63–72.

63. Crowley F, Mihalopoulos M, Gaglani S, et al. Prostate cancer in transgender women: considerations for screening, diagnosis and management. Br J Cancer 2023;128(2). https://doi.org/10.1038/s41416-022-01989-y.

64. Nik-Ahd F, Jarjour A, Figueiredo J, et al. Prostate-specific antigen screening in transgender patients. Eur Urol 2023;83(1). https://doi.org/10.1016/j.eururo.2022.09.007.

65. Weyers S, De Sutter P, Hoebeke S, et al. Gynaecological aspects of the treatment and follow-up of transsexual men and women. Facts Views Vis Obgyn 2010;2(1).

66. Nolan IT, Kuhner CJ, Dy GW. Demographic and temporal trends in transgender identities and gender confirming surgery. Transl Androl Urol 2019;8(3). https://doi.org/10.21037/tau.2019.04.09.

67. Safer JD, Coleman E, Feldman J, et al. Barriers to healthcare for transgender individuals. Curr Opin Endocrinol Diabetes Obes 2016;23(2). https://doi.org/10.1097/MED.0000000000000227.

Current State of Urology Residency Education on Caring for Transgender and Non-Binary Patients

R. Craig Sineath, MD, MPH[a],*, Finn Hennig, BS[b], Geolani W. Dy, MD[a]

KEYWORDS

- Transgender • Gender-affirming surgery • Urology • Resident education

KEY POINTS

- Educational content regarding urologic care for the transgender and nonbinary (TGNB) patients is limited but improving and is an important aspect of addressing urologic health disparities among TGNB communities.
- All urologists should be familiar with the general care of TGNB patients.
- Gender-affirming hormone therapy is a medical intervention that aligns secondary sexual characteristics with a person's gender identity.
- Gender affirming surgical care includes genital surgeries including vaginoplasty, phalloplasty, and metoidioplasty. All urologists should be familiar with these procedures and their respective complications.

INTRODUCTION

Urologists care for genitourinary conditions among all populations. Transgender and nonbinary (TGNB) patients are a population with unique urologic needs that are often overlooked in urologic training. TGNB people are those whose gender (a person's internal sense of how they fit in the world) differs from their sex assigned at birth (based on an assessment of their external genitalia).[1] Genderqueer, gender nonconforming, or nonbinary people are those who do not identify as gender on a binary scale (male/female) but as a spectrum between feminine and masculine.[1,2]

Recent studies estimate that up to 1% to 2% of the population identifies as TGNB,[3] with an estimated total size of 2 million transgender people in the United States.[4,5] TGNB people experience discrimination and stigma throughout all parts of life, including when accessing health care. This contributes to the many health disparities experienced by the TGNB population. TGNB people are more likely to experience sexual assault, poverty, unemployment, housing discrimination and homelessness, and are less likely to complete a high school education compared with their cisgender counterparts.[6–8] They are also more likely to live alone and not be married, a marker of social exclusion, which has been demonstrated to affect health outcomes.[6] TGNB patients are more likely to use tobacco and excessive alcohol, have low utilization of cancer screening, and have poor

Note: race/ethnicity denotes that both race and ethnicity were combined in this analysis but that race and ethnicity are distinctly different and not synonymous.

[a] Department of Urology, Oregon Health and Science University, 3303 South Bond Avenue Building 1, 10th Floor, Portland, OR 97239, USA; [b] Jacobs School of Medicine and Biomedical Sciences, University of Buffalo, 955 Main Street, Buffalo, NY 14203, USA

* Corresponding author.

E-mail address: sineath@ohsu.edu

urologic.theclinics.com

mental health outcomes.[9] An estimated 40% of TGNB people have attempted suicide, compared with only 4.6% of the general population.[7]

TGNB patients are less likely to access general health care in general due to experiences of transphobia, discrimination, health insurance policies, lack of ability to find employment, and the other social determinants of health previously described.[10] A Canadian study from 2018 that surveyed residents from various medical and surgical specialties showed that only 50% of urology residents surveyed thought that TGNB health care fell within their specialty, with 21% of these respondents stating they were uncomfortable seeing a transgender man about a general urology problem.[11] This same article demonstrated that some physicians may refuse to treat TGNB patients, citing conflict with personal religious beliefs or that caring for TGNB individuals is unethical.[11]

Contrary to this, several recent studies have shown that many health-care professionals and professional students exhibit comfort in treating TGNB patients but lack the knowledge in this specialized area.[12,13] A 2016 qualitative study interviewing 30 transgender patients and 11 physicians to evaluate how knowledge gaps can create barriers to care showed that almost all patient participants reported encounters with physicians who had significant gaps in their knowledge on treating transgender patients.[14] As a result, patients may be unable to access the care they need or are referred on to specialty centers with significant waitlists.

All urologists, regardless of subspecialty, are likely to see TGNB patients in their practice. TGNB patients often feel the burden of having to educate others, including providers, about TGNB health issues, and this directly affects the care they receive.[15] Urologic providers have a duty to be educated on caring for this population in a culturally competent manner to reduce these disparities in an already vulnerable population.

Beyond meeting the general urologic needs of TGNB patients, genital gender-affirming surgery and management of genitourinary complications has become a mainstay within urology. A recent survey of reconstructive urologists demonstrated that 75% of respondents thought that gender-affirming care should be a discipline within the Society of Genitourinary Reconstructive Surgeons.[16] With growing access to gender-affirming surgical care, all urologists must be educated on working with TGNB patients. This article overviews the current literature on teaching of care for TGNB patients within the urology residency curriculum, gives a brief overview of what urologists should know about working with TGNB patients and provides resources for learning more about this topic.

CURRENT STATE OF TEACHINGS WITHIN UROLOGY RESIDENCIES

Several recent studies have demonstrated the current state of teachings regarding gender-affirming care and working with TGNB patients within urology residency curriculums. In terms of the amount of material covered throughout urology residency, a recent study showed that programs only have an average of 1 hour of didactic teaching and 2 hours of clinical exposure, with 42% of programs having no didactic sessions on gender-affirming care.[17] There has been a demonstrated regional variation in the amount of TGNB surgical education within urology residencies, with programs in the west and northeast having a significantly higher exposure to this content within their curriculums compared with other areas of the country.[18] Geographic variation in availability of transcompetent providers and legislative barriers lead many TGNB patients to travel out of state to access gender-affirming surgical care.[19]

This lack of training is not due to a lack of interest in learning this subject. Of 400 urology residents recently surveyed, 80% indicated that exposure to gender-affirming care was important for their training.[18] Furthermore, another study demonstrated that 29% of urology residents plan on incorporating gender-affirming care into their practice after graduation.[11]

There are barriers to including TGNB-specific material within urology residency curricula. Some barriers that have been identified include lack of educational materials, lack of faculty expertise, time and cost constraints, and challenges in recruiting and compensating TGNB guest speakers.[20]

Improving knowledge in gender-affirming urologic care is not only important for trainees but also for those who have completed training, particularly faculty within urology residency programs. Program directors' attitudes toward gender-affirming care have been linked to the amount of this material is taught to urology residents.[17] Faculty development is critical to allowing those with power to identify gaps in their knowledge and model positive professional behavior for their learners.[15]

Training programs have a responsibility to teach this and ensure adequate and inclusive access to care for this marginalized population. This fits with the Accreditation Council for Graduate Medical Education's requirement that trainees should effectively work with patients from a broad range of cultural and socioeconomic backgrounds.[21] The American Urologic Association (AUA) has made strides in this area with the inclusion of gender-affirming care within the core curriculum.

The remainder of this review focuses on general concepts that every urologist should know and consider when working with TGNB patients.

WHAT DOES EVERY UROLOGIST NEED TO KNOW ABOUT CARING FOR TGNB PATIENTS?
Definitions and Terminology

Urologists often work with patients in sensitive situations given the inherent nature of treating disorders of the genitourinary system. This is increasingly complex when working individuals who may have dysphoria around their genitalia and have likely been subject to discrimination and transphobia in health-care settings.[7] When a TGNB patient presents to a urologist, even with a simple complaint not related to their gender dysphoria, it is important for urologists to know how to correctly address TGNB patients in a sensitive and appropriate manner.

First, it is important for providers to use the correct and appropriate names and pronouns (eg, she/her, he/him, they/them, or others). Electronic medical systems have often not been updated to include chosen name and pronouns and rather present legal name and sex to providers before they meet the patient. Intake forms and electronic medical records that do not include items to capture transgender identity can make this population feel invisible and is an added barrier to providers appropriately addressing their patients.[15] The simple task of including gender and pronouns on an intake form can be an excellent tool that allows health-care team members to address each patient in a correct and culturally sensitive manner, improving the patient–provider relationship. If not provided on an intake form, clinicians may elicit this information by asking, "Which pronouns do you use?" We recommend including chosen name and pronouns, sex assigned at birth, and gender. Physicians should also advocate for their hospital system to update the electronic medical system to be inclusive of this information. Pronouns should be documented in notes because this is an easy way to communicate with other providers in the health-care system to ensure they are appropriately addressing the patient.[22] In all clinical documentation, patients should be referred to by their chosen name and pronouns.

Additionally, there are actions a clinic or health-care space can integrate that ensure TGNB patients feel safe and welcomed into the space, improving their likelihood to seek care and return for follow-up. Front desk staff are the first contact with patients and can set the tone for their visit.

Thus, it is critical that they are trained to appropriately address the patients in a nonjudgmental manner with their correct name and pronouns. Additionally, it is important to ensure that transgender patients have the facilities to take care of their basic needs (ie, bathrooms). These should be marked as either gender neutral or with a sign indicating that a person may choose the men's or women's bathroom based on their own personal preference.[1] Limiting stress and discrimination throughout the visit will improve the patient and physician relationship and make the patient more comfortable. This is especially important in the field of urology where we often must examine the sensitive areas, and most of these patients already have dysphoria around their genitals.

Given TGNB patients' history of discrimination and trauma, especially when accessing health care, enacting trauma-informed care principles is essential in gender-affirming care. Using a trauma-informed care model actively aims to reduce the retraumatization of patients and prevents triggering painful memories of earlier traumatic events.[23] Principles of trauma-informed care include approaching care through a patient-centered manner (ensuring physical and psychological safety of the patient), understanding the health effects of the experienced trauma and how this may play into the patient–provider relationship (ie, earlier negative experiences in health care leading to distrust of providers and the medical system), engaging interprofessional and community collaboration (ie, through mental health providers, patient advocates, and so forth), and understanding and reflecting on your own biases and how this may play into how you treat a patient.[24] The Substance Abuse and Mental Health Services Administration has released key principles of trauma-informed care, which are as follows[1]: safety[2]; trustworthiness and transparency[3]; peer support[4]; collaboration and mutuality[5]; empowerment, voice, and choice;[6] and cultural, historical, and gender issues.[23] Having a basic understanding of trauma-informed care principles can greatly influence care provided.

When a TGNB patient presents to a urologist for care, it is important to take a culturally sensitive surgical history and organ inventory to ensure appropriate diagnoses, risk factors, and screening examinations can be performed based on the present anatomy. This means gathering and documenting information on the patient's genital anatomy and prior surgical procedures independent of their gender identity, assigned sex, or preferred pronouns such as whether a patient has a prostate, vagina, cervix, uterus, ovaries, testes, and so forth.[25,26]

Additionally, it is important to know the changes in anatomy and how these may affect a treatment plan. The genital examination may be an especially triggering event for TGNB patients given their potential genital dysphoria and increased likelihood of prior sexual assault relative to the general population.[27] Performing a sensitive physical examination without appropriate care can cause harm to the patient and the patient–physician relationship. Trauma-informed care principles for completing the physical examination include preparing the patient for the examination, warning the patient before touch, involving the patient in the examination, performing the examination in their preferred position, asking about preferred language for genitalia (ie, some transmasculine patients may prefer the word "canal" instead of "vagina" because vagina can be considered gendered), and ensuring a chaperone is present.[22]

Additionally, when developing new clinical care pathways for this population, it is crucial to have community engagement and partnership. Developing positive community relationships between medical personnel and the TGB community through community engagement is one way that could improve TGNB community access to health care and improve their trust in the medical system.[15] This also helps the organization further understand this population's unique needs and ensure they are considered.

Overview of Gender Affirming Hormone Therapy

Gender-affirming hormone therapy (GAHT) is a medical intervention that aligns secondary sexual characteristics with a person's gender identity. GAHT is typically prescribed by a patient's primary care doctor or endocrinologist. Feminizing hormone therapy typically consists of the patient taking an estrogen and an antiandrogen such as spironolactone or 5-alpha reductase inhibitor. Once a patient has undergone a gender-affirming bilateral orchiectomy, they can often stop taking the antiandrogen medication and often reduce their estrogen dosage, and therefore should follow up with their hormone prescriber to update their regimen.[1] Masculinizing hormone therapy consists of patients taking testosterone in various forms, which urologists are very comfortable prescribing for cisgender men with symptoms of low testosterone.[1]

Gonodotropic releasing hormone agonist such as leuprolide can be prescribed as puberty blockers (PB) for prepubertal patients who identify as TGNB. These medications allow patients to further explore their gender identity and expression while preventing the permanent and often dysphoria-inducing secondary sexual characteristic changes of masculinizing or feminizing puberty such as voice deepening, facial hair development, thyroid cartilage growth, or breast growth and have been demonstrated to improve psychological well-being and reduce suicidal ideation.[28–30] One study among TGNB youth showed that starting a patient on gender-affirming hormone therapy (GAHT) or PB significantly reduces depression (60% lower odds) and suicidality (73% lower odds).[31] These can reduce a person's potential need for surgical procedures and other treatments such as hair removal and voice training later in life and have been demonstrated to be safe in short-term studies, and long-term studies are currently being conducted.[32,33] Patients with potential interest in vaginoplasty should be counseled that these can lead to genital hypoplasia necessitating potential need for the use of nongenital tissue (ie, skin grafting or peritoneal flaps) for vaginal canal creation.

Overview of Gender Affirming Surgeries

Gender-affirming surgery includes a broad range of procedures and may be an important part of the transition process for some but not all TGNB people. Access to surgical transition for those who seek it reduces suicide risk and can greatly improves an individual's quality of life.[34,35] The World Professional Association for Transgender Health (WPATH) has recently released version 8 of the standards of care guidelines for providers to use when offering patients care for medical and surgical transition. Criteria for surgery include sustained gender incongruence, capacity for consent, an assessment of mental health and physical conditions that could influence the outcomes of surgery, and stability for a minimum of 6 months of hormone therapy if hormone therapy is within the patient's goals and not medically contraindicated.[36] Fertility options must be discussed before gonadectomy.[36] The new guidelines have shifted toward a shared decision-making model and no longer mention a requirement for letters from a mental health provider for gender-affirming surgery due to this being a major barrier to access to care for many patients.

Gender-Affirming Surgery, complications, and Concerns for Treating General Urologic Disorders

Many gender-affirming surgeries are complex reconstructive surgeries of the urogenital system. As such, they innately have complications that urologists should be familiar with as patients may present to any health center for acute or long-term management.

Phalloplasty and metoidioplasty

Genital gender-affirming surgeries for individuals assigned female at birth can include vaginectomy, hysterectomy, scrotoplasty, metoidioplasty (lengthening of the virilized clitoris, with or without urethral lengthening), and phalloplasty (creation of a phallus with or without urethral lengthening, with or without placement of a penile prosthesis). Those who have undergone metoidioplasty or phalloplasty are encouraged to have lifelong urologic follow-up; those who have undergone vaginoplasty should follow-up with their primary surgeon, or for longer term care, with a primary care physician or gynecologist who is knowledgeable about the patient's long-term surgical maintenance needs.[36]

After urethral lengthening in phalloplasty, the urethra can be described in 3 parts. There is the native urethra, the perineal urethra, or pars fixa (from the perineal scrotal junction to the neophallus), and the penile urethra.[37] Common complications after urethral lengthening include fistula and stricture.[37] Urinary fistulas have been described to occur in 15% to 70% and strictures between 14% and 52% of patients who undergo phalloplasty with urethral lengthening and may not require surgical management because many resolve spontaneously.[38] Strictures, however, do typically require treatment given risks of acute or long-term lower urinary tract obstruction including increased risk for urinary tract infections, development of lower urinary tract symptoms such as urgency and frequency, and damage to the bladder. We describe acute management of urinary retention below. For more definitive treatment, patients should be referred to a reconstructive urologist who has experience managing urethral complications after genital gender-affirming surgery.

Orchiectomy, vaginoplasty, and vulvoplasty

Genital gender-affirming surgeries for individuals assigned male at birth may include bilateral simple orchiectomy, scrotectomy, vaginoplasty, and vulvoplasty (external reconstruction without a neovaginal canal). Bilateral simple orchiectomy is a procedure that can be performed by any urologist. This procedure has been demonstrated have many significant benefits for TGNB patients including the ability to discontinue antiandrogens which often have negative side effect, lowering the dose of estrogen needed (usually by about 50%), the ability to conceal their genitalia or "tuck" more comfortably, and it affirms their gender. (Core curriculum – CC) Performing this procedure on its own does not preclude patients from undergoing a vaginoplasty later in life. Gender-affirming orchiectomy should be done

with a midline scrotal incision to preserve blood supply for future potential surgeries and removing the spermatic cord to the peritoneal reflection to reduce bulging in the area.

Vaginoplasty typically involves partial penectomy, clitoroplasty, labiaplasty, urethral meatus repositioning, and creation of an internal vaginal canal. The vaginal canal can be developed from a variety of means including penile skin inversion and scrotal skin graft, peritoneal flaps, or intestinal transposition.

Rectoneovaginal fistula, vesiconeovaginal fistula, vaginal stenosis with resultant neovaginal abscess, and neovaginal perforation are rare but can be complications of vaginoplasty.[39] Rectovaginal fistula most often occurs if a rectal injury is made at the time of surgery during the canal dissection.[40]

More common postoperative events include labial wound separation or superficial skin necrosis, especially in the posterior introitus where there is often the most tension at the completion of reconstruction, among patients who have undergone vaginoplasty and vulvoplasty. These are usually treated with simply with wound dressing changes; patients with vaginoplasty must continue vaginal dilation in the early postoperative period despite wound breakdown. Granulation tissue may develop in the first few months after surgery, at the external vulva or within the vaginal canal and can be managed with silver nitrate.[41]

Vaginal stenosis occurs in about 10% of patients,[42] although these rates may be underestimated due to lack of longitudinal follow-up in many vaginoplasty studies. To prevent this, patients must perform lifelong vaginal dilation. In the immediate postoperative phase, most surgeons require that patients dilate 3 to 4 times per day until they reach their goal size dilator without difficulty, and eventually they can wean down with the goal of eventually just dilating 1 to 2 times per week to maintain depth and width.[41] These recommendations may vary by surgical technique and surgeon practice.

Patients who have undergone robotic peritoneal flap vaginoplasty can have intra-abdominal complications associated with any robotic surgery that all urologists are familiar with. These complications are rare but include small bowel obstruction, hernias, pelvic abscess, and rectal injury.[43–45] Other rare but urgent complications include peritoneal flap dehiscence, herniation, or evisceration.

Troubleshooting general urologic concerns

Urologists treat all disorders of the genitourinary system including nephrolithiasis, cancer, infections, and lower urinary tract symptoms. TGNB patients may have anatomy that is altered from their natal anatomy, and when a TGNB patient presents with concern that may need treatment, a urologist must be able to gather information on earlier surgical procedures and current anatomy, and then navigate how this will affect surgical planning.

Patients who have undergone vaginoplasty or vulvoplasty may also present with complaints of their urinary stream. A spraying stream may be associated with obstructing skin or meatal stenosis and occurs in 6% to 33% of patients.[40,46] This can be treated with a simple meatoplasty or a Y-V skin advancement flap.

If a patient requires a Foley catheter, some may find this difficult to place in patients who have undergone gender-affirming genital surgeries with alterations to the native urethra. If the provider is having difficulty finding this, they can ask the patient to point to their urethral meatus because they will likely be familiar with their anatomy. In patients who have undergone vaginoplasty or vulvoplasty, the urethra can be found beneath the clitoris and just above the vaginal canal, if a canal is present. If there is concern for a stricture, a flexible cystoscope or ureteroscope can be used to get a wire across the urethra for dilation.

In patients who have undergone phalloplasty with urethral lengthening, great care should be taken when placing a Foley. Unless known urethral stricture or other complications are present, we recommend a first attempt at catheterization with a 16Fr coude catheter and gentle pressure; if any resistance is met, there should be a very low threshold for using a scope to place the catheter to ensure the reconstructed urethra is not injured and that the catheter tip is being directed into the true bladder neck and lumen rather than a posterior pit corresponding to the prior vaginal canal. In those who have undergone phalloplasty or metoidioplasty with urethral lengthening, we recommend using a flexible cystoscope, pediatric flexible cystoscope, or a flexible ureteroscope to avoid injury to the urethra.[41] If the provider is unable to access a bladder for drainage in this way, a suprapubic tube should be placed in the event of acute urinary retention. In a patient who has had a recent urethral lengthening procedure, a suprapubic tube may be a safer option rather than cystoscopy given their anastomoses are still healing and may be at risk of being injured with a cystoscope. These same principles should be applied with accessing the bladder for other endoscopic surgeries including laser lithotripsy and transurethral resection of bladder tumors.

Voiding dysfunction TGNB patients experience high rates voiding dysfunction. This is in part due to their experience of harassment and violence and lack of safe restroom access. In a large survey conducted by the National Center for Transgender equality, 9% of participants were denied access to a restroom in the past year, 12% were verbally harassed when accessing a restroom, and 59% indicated they avoided using public restrooms due to fear of harassment.[7] Bathroom avoidance has been linked to increase in overactive bladder symptoms and stress urinary incontinence.[47] This, along with an increased risk of being diagnosed with anxiety disorders, can contribute to many urinary symptoms including voiding dysfunction and pelvic floor disorders.

TGNB patients may present with benign prostatic hyperplasia despite being on estrogen and androgen blockade, particularly if these were started later in life. If these patients are indicated for an outlet procedure, their goals regarding additional vaginoplasty or vulvoplasty should be considered. Those who undergo an outlet procedure may have compromise of the bladder neck and subsequent vaginoplasty with canal dissection may lead to florid incontinence due to external sphincter disruption, with no reliable option for surgical correction. Vulvoplasty is a safer alternative to reduce incontinence risk after bladder outlet procedures, however, may not meet a patient's surgical transition goals. Long-term urinary outcomes of vaginoplasty and vulvoplasty after surgical interventions for BPH are understudied; in the meantime, we recommend that urologists consider alternative procedures to transurethral resection of the prostate such as UroLift.

WHERE CAN YOU LEARN MORE?

A literature review published in 2020 identified resources being used for training in TGNB health care, including continuing medical education (CME) courses, online web module, and interdisciplinary interventions, all of which were demonstrated to improve competency in providing care for this marginalized population.[48] They highlighted 7 professional societies that offered online CME material on TGNB health including the American Medical Association, the American College of Physicians, the Endocrine Society, the American Academy of Otolaryngology—Head and Neck Surgery, the American Society of Plastic Surgeons, the American College of Obstetricians and Gynecologists, and the AUA.

AUA's Core Curriculum now includes a section on the "Care of Transgender and Gender Non-Conforming Patients" with 4 articles covering

Table 1
Overview of terminology

Term	Definition	Example
Gender dysphoria	Distress that results from an incongruence of one's gender identity and their sex assigned at birth	
Pronouns	How a person refers to themselves	He/him, she/her, they/them, and so forth
Gender neutral	Not referring to being a man or woman	They/them are considered gender-neutral pronouns. Gender neutral bathrooms are labeled to where someone of any gender can use
Organ inventory	A surgical history that takes into account which organs are still present and may	Presence of cervix, uterus, ovaries, or prostate
GAHT	Medications that align secondary sexual characteristics with a patient's gender	Testosterone, estrogen, spironolactone, and so forth
Masculinizing gender-affirming surgery	Surgeries that remove feminine or add masculine secondary sexual characteristics	Mastectomy, metoidioplasty, and phalloplasty
Feminizing gender-affirming surgery	Surgeries that remove masculine or add feminine secondary sexual characteristics	Breast implants, vaginoplasty, and vulvoplasty

gender-affirming hormone therapy, medical management and presurgery preparation, masculinizing and feminizing genital gender-affirming surgery, and general urologic care for the TGNB patient.[41] The AUA course, "Genital Gender Affirming Surgery for Transgender Patients" (Update Series Volume 36, 2017) provides an overview of affirming transgender terminology, surgical options, postoperative management, and accepted care guidelines.[49] Additionally, the most recent 2022 Update Series offers "A Urologist's Guide to Caring for the Transfeminine Patient," which provides insight on how to provide culturally competent care for this population as well as addressing common urologic issues affecting TGNB patients.[50] The National LGBTQIA + Health Education Center at The Fenway Institute also offers CME-accredited webinars covering a wide range of topics including surgical care, trauma-informed care, hormone therapy, and reproductive health with regards to the TGNB community.[51]

The University of California San Francisco (UCSF) guidelines also provide a comprehensive guide to TGNB care ranging from basic terminology to urology-specific topics.[1] Sections of note include prostate and testicular cancer considerations in transgender women, pelvic and scrotal pain assessment and management, as well as overview and postoperative considerations for vaginoplasty, phalloplasty, and metoidioplasty (**Table 1**).

To help obstetrics and gynecology (OB-GYN) residents meet Council on Resident Education in Obstetrics and Gynecology (CREOG) objectives related to caring for TGNB patients, physicians from Michigan Medicine collaborated to develop 5 approximately 15-minute modules.[52] These modules cover treatment, preventative care, and common gynecologic concerns for TGNB individuals. A unique aspect to their training is a module specifically created to address health records, billing, and insurance in TGNB medicine.

Many health professionals look to the WPATH for guidance in caring for TGNB patients.[36] The recent updates to these standards of care expand on the categories of medically necessary surgical interventions to include facial surgery and gonadectomy, which many current health-care plans regard as cosmetic and therefore do not cover. Additionally, the length of hormone therapy before GGAS has also been made more individually based with a 6-month recommendation instead of the prior 12 months.

SUMMARY

Educational content regarding urologic care for the TGNB patients is limited but improving and is an important aspect of addressing urologic health disparities among TGNB communities. As the field of gender-affirming care grows, many residents and urologists see gender-affirming surgery as a mainstay within urology.

All urologists should be familiar with the general care of TGNB patients. This includes knowing how to speak with TGNB patients in an appropriate and nonstigmatizing manner, using trauma-informed care principles for clinical encounters, adequately and sensitively taking an organ inventory to ensure appropriate diagnoses and treatment options are considered, and understanding basic principles of genital gender-affirming surgeries, including potential urologic complications.

CLINICS CARE POINTS

- All urologists are likely to see transgender and non-binary patients in their practice and should be familiar with complications and their management after genital gender-affirming surgery.

- Sensitive physical examinations should be conducted utilizing trauma-informed care principles.

- Gender-affirming hormone therapy is a medical intervention that aligns secondary sexual characteristics with a person's gender identity.

- Gender-affirming surgery includes a broad range of procedures. Genital gender-affirming surgeries that include the urogenital system include vulvoplasty, vaginoplasty, metoidioplasty, and phalloplasty.

REFERENCES

1. UCSF Gender Affirming Health Program, Department of Family and Community Medicine, University of California San Francisco. Guidelines for the Primary and Gender-Affirming Care of Transgender and Gender Nonbinary People; 2nd edition. Deutsch M.B., ed. June 2016. Available at: transcare.ucsf.edu/guidelines.
2. Lagos D. Looking at Population Health Beyond "Male" and "Female": Implications of Transgender Identity and Gender Nonconformity for Population Health. Demography 2018;55(6):2097–117.
3. Sexual Orientation and Gender Identity in the Household Pulse Survey. Unites States Census Bureau. 2021.
4. Nolan IT, Kuhner CJ, Dy GW. Demographic and temporal trends in transgender identities and gender confirming surgery. Transl Androl Urol 2019;8(3):184–90.
5. Flores AR, Herman JL, Gates GJ, et al. How many adults identify as transgender in the United States. Los Angeles, CA: The WIlliams Institute; 2016.
6. Fredriksen Goldsen KI, Romanelli M, Hoy-Ellis CP, et al. economic and social disparities among transgender women, transgender men and transgender nonbinary adults: Results from a population-based study. Prev Med 2022;156:106988.
7. James SE, Herman JL, Rankin S, et al. The report of the 2015 transgender survey. Washington, DC: National Center for Transgender Equality; 2016.
8. Douglass KM, Polcari A, Najjar N, et al. Health Care for the Homeless Transgender Community: Psychiatric Services and Transition Care at a Student-Run Clinic. J Health Care Poor Underserved 2018;29(3):940–8.
9. Domogauer J, Cantor T, Quinn G, et al. Disparities in cancer screenings for sexual and gender minorities. Curr Probl Cancer 2022;46(5):100858.
10. Gonzales G, Henning-Smith C. Barriers to Care Among Transgender and Gender Nonconforming Adults. Milbank Q 2017;95(4):726–48.
11. Coutin A, Wright S, Li C, et al. Missed opportunities: are residents prepared to care for transgender patients? A study of family medicine, psychiatry, endocrinology, and urology residents. Can Med Educ J 2018;9(3):e41–55.
12. Vasudevan A, García AD, Hart BG, et al. Health Professions Students' Knowledge, Skills, and Attitudes Toward Transgender Healthcare. J Community Health 2022;47(6):981–9.
13. Kelly-Schuette K, Little A, Davis AT, et al. Transgender Surgery: Perspectives Across Levels of Training in Medical and Surgical Specialties. Transgend Health 2021;6(4):217–23.
14. McPhail D, Rountree-James M, Whetter I. Addressing gaps in physician knowledge regarding transgender health and healthcare through medical education. Can Med Educ J 2016;7(2):e70–8.
15. Noonan EJ, Sawning S, Combs R, et al. Engaging the Transgender Community to Improve Medical Education and Prioritize Healthcare Initiatives. Teach Learn Med 2018;30(2):119–32.
16. Sukumar S, Pijush DB, Brandes SB. Gender Affirming Surgery Experience and Exposure among Reconstructive Urologists. Urology Practice 2020;7(3):234–40.
17. Morrison SD, Dy GW, Chong HJ, et al. Transgender-Related Education in Plastic Surgery and Urology Residency Programs. J Grad Med Educ 2017;9(2):178–83.
18. Dy GW, Osbun NC, Morrison SD, et al. Exposure to and Attitudes Regarding Transgender Education Among Urology Residents. J Sex Med 2016;13(10):1466–72.
19. Downing J, Holt SK, Cunetta M, et al. Spending and Out-of-Pocket Costs for Genital Gender-Affirming

Surgery in the US. JAMA Surg 2022;157(9): 799–806.

20. van Heesewijk J, Kent A, van de Grift TC, et al. Transgender health content in medical education: a theory-guided systematic review of current training practices and implementation barriers & facilitators. Adv Health Sci Educ Theory Pract 2022;27(3): 817–46.

21. Balbona J, Patel T. The Hidden Curriculum: Strategies for Preparing Residents for Practice. Curr Urol Rep 2020;21(10):39.

22. Scull D, Chung PH, Dugi D, et al. Creating a Gender-Affirming Environment for Urologic Care. AUA News 2021;26(4).

23. Substance Abuse and Mental Health Services Administration. SAMHSA's Concept of Trauma and Guidance for a Trauma-Informed Approach. HHS Publication No. In: (SMA)14-4884. Rockville, MD: Substance Abuse and Mental Health Services Administration; 2014.

24. Raja S, Hasnain M, Hoersch M, et al. Trauma Informed Care in Medicine: Current Knowledge and Future Research Directions. Fam Community Health 2015;38:216–26.

25. Rosendale N, Goldman S, Ortiz GM, et al. Acute Clinical Care for Transgender Patients: A Review. JAMA Intern Med 2018;178(11):1535–43.

26. Driver L, Egan DJ, Hsiang E, et al. Block by block: Building on our knowledge to better care for LGBTQIA+ patients. AEM Educ Train 2022;6(Suppl 1). S57–s63.

27. Newcomb ME, Hill R, Buehler K, et al. High Burden of Mental Health Problems, Substance Use, Violence, and Related Psychosocial Factors in Transgender, Non-Binary, and Gender Diverse Youth and Young Adults. Arch Sex Behav 2020;49(2): 645–59.

28. Schulmeister C, Millington K, Kaufman M, et al. Growth in Transgender/Gender-Diverse Youth in the First Year of Treatment With Gonadotropin-Releasing Hormone Agonists. J Adolesc Health 2022;70(1):108–13.

29. Turban JL, King D, Carswell JM, et al. Pubertal Suppression for Transgender Youth and Risk of Suicidal Ideation. Pediatrics 2020;145(2).

30. van de Grift TC, van Gelder ZJ, Mullender MG, et al. Timing of Puberty Suppression and Surgical Options for Transgender Youth. Pediatrics 2020;146(5).

31. Tordoff DM, Wanta JW, Collin A, et al. Mental Health Outcomes in Transgender and Nonbinary Youths Receiving Gender-Affirming Care. JAMA Netw Open 2022;5(2):e220978.

32. Olson-Kennedy J, Chan YM, Garofalo R, et al. Impact of Early Medical Treatment for Transgender Youth: Protocol for the Longitudinal, Observational Trans Youth Care Study. JMIR Res Protoc 2019; 8(7):e14434.

33. Lee JY, Rosenthal SM. Gender-Affirming Care of Transgender and Gender-Diverse Youth: Current Concepts. Annu Rev Med 2023;74:107–16.

34. Bauer GR, Scheim AI, Pyne J, et al. Intervenable factors associated with suicide risk in transgender persons: a respondent driven sampling study in Ontario, Canada. BMC Publ Health 2015;15:525.

35. Padula WV, Heru S, Campbell JD. Societal Implications of Health Insurance Coverage for Medically Necessary Services in the U.S. Transgender Population: A Cost-Effectiveness Analysis. J Gen Intern Med 2016;31(4):394–401.

36. Coleman E, Radix AE, Bouman WP, et al. Standards of Care for the Health of Transgender and Gender Diverse People, Version 8. Int J Transgend Health 2022;23(Suppl 1). S1–s259.

37. Veerman H, de Rooij FPW, Al-Tamimi M, et al. Functional Outcomes and Urological Complications after Genital Gender Affirming Surgery with Urethral Lengthening in Transgender Men. J Urol 2020; 204(1):104–9.

38. Santucci RA. Urethral Complications After Transgender Phalloplasty: Strategies to Treat Them and Minimize Their Occurrence. Clin Anat 2018;31(2):187–90.

39. Gaither TW, Awad MA, Osterberg EC, et al. Postoperative Complications following Primary Penile Inversion Vaginoplasty among 330 Male-to-Female Transgender Patients. J Urol 2018;199(3):760–5.

40. Horbach SE, Bouman MB, Smit JM, et al. Outcome of Vaginoplasty in Male-to-Female Transgenders: A Systematic Review of Surgical Techniques. J Sex Med 2015;12(6):1499–512.

41. AUA Urology Core Curriculum: AUA University; 2023 Available at: https://auau.auanet.org/core. Accessed February 18, 2023.

42. Dreher PC, Edwards D, Hager S, et al. Complications of the neovagina in male-to-female transgender surgery: A systematic review and meta-analysis with discussion of management. Clin Anat 2018;31(2):191–9.

43. Dy GW, Jun MS, Blasdel G, et al. Outcomes of Gender Affirming Peritoneal Flap Vaginoplasty Using the Da Vinci Single Port Versus Xi Robotic Systems. Eur Urol 2021;79(5):676–83.

44. Jacoby A, Maliha S, Granieri MA, et al. Robotic Davydov Peritoneal Flap Vaginoplasty for Augmentation of Vaginal Depth in Feminizing Vaginoplasty. J Urol 2019;201(6):1171–6.

45. Acar O, Sofer L, Dobbs RW, et al. Single Port and Multiport Approaches for Robotic Vaginoplasty With the Davydov Technique. Urology 2020;138:166–73.

46. Hadj-Moussa M, Ohl DA, Kuzon WM Jr. Feminizing Genital Gender-Confirmation Surgery. Sex Med Rev 2018;6(3):457–68.e2.

47. Reynolds WS, Kowalik C, Kaufman MR, et al. Women's Perceptions of Public Restrooms and the Relationships with Toileting Behaviors and Bladder

Symptoms: A Cross-Sectional Study. J Urol 2020; 204(2):310–5.

48. Nolan IT, Blasdel G, Dubin SN, et al. Current State of Transgender Medical Education in the United States and Canada: Update to a Scoping Review. J Med Educ Curric Dev 2020;7. 2382120520934813.

49. Garcia MM, Christopher NA. Update Series Lesson 5: Genital Gender Affirming Surgery for Transgender Patients. In: Update Series37. AUA University; 2017.

50. Butler C, Dugi D. Update Series Lesson 3: A Urologist's Guide to Caring for the Transfeminine Patient. In: Update Series41. AUA University; 2022.

51. Learning Resources — Transgender Health: National LGBTQIA+ Health Education Center: A Program of the Fenway Institute; Available at: https://www.lgbtqiahealtheducation.org/resources/in/transgender-health/. Accessed February 18, 2023.

52. Improving Ob-Gyn Care for Transgender and Non-Binary Individuals The American College of Obstetricians and Gynecologists 2022 Available from: https://www.acog.org/education-and-events/creog/curriculum-resources/additional-curricular-resources/transgender-health-care. Accessed February 18, 2023.

UNITED STATES POSTAL SERVICE ®

Statement of Ownership, Management, and Circulation
(All Periodicals Publications Except Requester Publications)

1. Publication Title: UROLOGIC CLINICS OF NORTH AMERICA

2. Publication Number: 000 – 711

3. Filing Date: 9/18/2023

4. Issue Frequency: FEB, MAY, AUG, NOV

5. Number of Issues Published Annually: 4

6. Annual Subscription Price: $415.00

7. Complete Mailing Address of Known Office of Publication (Not printed) (Street, city, county, state, and ZIP+4®)
ELSEVIER INC.
230 Park Avenue, Suite 800
New York, NY 10169

Contact Person: Malathi Samayan
Telephone (Include area code): 91-44-4299-4507

8. Complete Mailing Address of Headquarters or General Business Office of Publisher (Not printer)
ELSEVIER INC.
230 Park Avenue, Suite 800
New York, NY 10169

9. Full Names and Complete Mailing Addresses of Publisher, Editor, and Managing Editor (Do not leave blank)

Publisher (Name and complete mailing address)
Dolores Meloni, ELSEVIER INC.
1600 JOHN F KENNEDY BLVD. SUITE 1600
PHILADELPHIA, PA 19103-2899

Editor (Name and complete mailing address)
KERRY HOLLAND, ELSEVIER INC.
1600 JOHN F KENNEDY BLVD. SUITE 1600
PHILADELPHIA, PA 19103-2899

Managing Editor (Name and complete mailing address)
PATRICK MANLEY, ELSEVIER INC.
1600 JOHN F KENNEDY BLVD. SUITE 1600
PHILADELPHIA, PA 19103-2899

10. Owner (Do not leave blank. If the publication is owned by a corporation, give the name and address of the corporation immediately followed by the names and addresses of all stockholders owning or holding 1 percent or more of the total amount of stock. If not owned by a corporation, give the names and addresses of the individual owners. If owned by a partnership or other unincorporated firm, give its name and address as well as those of each individual owner. If the publication is published by a nonprofit organization, give its name and address.)

Full Name	Complete Mailing Address
WHOLLY OWNED SUBSIDIARY OF REED/ELSEVIER, US HOLDINGS	1600 JOHN F KENNEDY BLVD. SUITE 1600 PHILADELPHIA, PA 19103-2899

11. Known Bondholders, Mortgagees, and Other Security Holders Owning or Holding 1 Percent or More of Total Amount of Bonds, Mortgages, or Other Securities. If none, check box ☐ None

Full Name	Complete Mailing Address
N/A	

12. Tax Status (For completion by nonprofit organizations authorized to mail at nonprofit rates) (Check one)
The purpose, function, and nonprofit status of this organization and the exempt status for federal income tax purposes:
☒ Has Not Changed During Preceding 12 Months
☐ Has Changed During Preceding 12 Months (Publisher must submit explanation of change with this statement)

PS Form 3526, July 2014 [Page 1 of 4 (see instructions page 4)] PSN 7530-01-000-9931 PRIVACY NOTICE: See our privacy policy on www.usps.com.

---

13. Publication Title: UROLOGIC CLINICS OF NORTH AMERICA

14. Issue Date for Circulation Data Below: AUGUST 2023

15. Extent and Nature of Circulation

		Average No. Copies Each Issue During Preceding 12 Months	No. Copies of Single Issue Published Nearest to Filing Date
a. Total Number of Copies (Net press run)		164	148
b. Paid Circulation (By Mail and Outside the Mail)	(1) Mailed Outside-County Paid Subscriptions Stated on PS Form 3541 (Include paid distribution above nominal rate, advertiser's proof copies, and exchange copies)	89	73
	(2) Mailed In-County Paid Subscriptions Stated on PS Form 3541 (Include paid distribution above nominal rate, advertiser's proof copies, and exchange copies)	0	0
	(3) Paid Distribution Outside the Mails Including Sales Through Dealers and Carriers, Street Vendors, Counter Sales, and Other Paid Distribution Outside USPS®	63	63
	(4) Paid Distribution by Other Classes of Mail Through the USPS (e.g., First-Class Mail®)	9	9
c. Total Paid Distribution (Sum of 15b (1), (2), (3), and (4))		161	145
d. Free or Nominal Rate Distribution (By Mail and Outside the Mail)	(1) Free or Nominal Rate Outside-County Copies Included on PS Form 3541	3	3
	(2) Free or Nominal Rate In-County Copies Included on PS Form 3541	0	0
	(3) Free or Nominal Rate Copies Mailed at Other Classes Through the USPS (e.g., First-Class Mail)	0	0
	(4) Free or Nominal Rate Distribution Outside the Mail (Carriers or other means)	0	0
e. Total Free or Nominal Rate Distribution (Sum of 15d (1), (2), (3) and (4))		3	3
f. Total Distribution (Sum of 15c and 15e)		164	148
g. Copies not Distributed (See Instructions to Publishers #4 (page 83))		0	0
h. Total (Sum of 15f and g)		164	148
i. Percent Paid (15c divided by 15f times 100)		98.17%	97.97%

* If you are claiming electronic copies, go to line 16 on page 3. If you are not claiming electronic copies, skip to line 17 on page 3.

PS Form 3526, July 2014 (Page 2 of 4)

16. Electronic Copy Circulation

	Average No. Copies Each Issue During Preceding 12 Months	No. Copies of Single Issue Published Nearest to Filing Date
a. Paid Electronic Copies		
b. Total Paid Print Copies (Line 15c) + Paid Electronic Copies (Line 16a)		
c. Total Print Distribution (Line 15f) + Paid Electronic Copies (Line 16a)		
d. Percent Paid (Both Print & Electronic Copies) (16b divided by 16c × 100)		

☒ I certify that 50% of all my distributed copies (electronic and print) are paid above a nominal price.

17. Publication of Statement of Ownership

☒ If the publication is a general publication, publication of this statement is required. Will be printed in the NOVEMBER 2023 issue of this publication. ☐ Publication not required.

18. Signature and Title of Editor, Publisher, Business Manager, or Owner

Malathi Samayan - Distribution Controller

Malathi Samayan

Date: 9/18/2023

I certify that all information furnished on this form is true and complete. I understand that anyone who furnishes false or misleading information on this form or who omits material or information requested on the form may be subject to criminal sanctions (including fines and imprisonment) and/or civil sanctions (including civil penalties).

PS Form 3526, July 2014 (Page 3 of 4) PRIVACY NOTICE: See our privacy policy on www.usps.com.

Printed and bound by CPI Group (UK) Ltd, Croydon, CR0 4YY

08/05/2025

01864748-0014